SOAP
for
Pediatrics

Look for other books in this series!

SOAP for Obstetrics and Gynecology

SOAP for Emergency Medicine

SOAP for Family Medicine

SOAP for Internal Medicine

SOAP for Urology

SOAP for Neurology

SOAP
for
Pediatrics

Michael A. Polisky, MD
Resident, Internal Medicine-Pediatrics
Los Angeles County-USC Medical Center
Los Angeles, California

Breck Nichols, MD, MPH
Resident, Internal Medicine-Pediatrics
Los Angeles County-USC Medical Center
Los Angeles, California

Series Editor:
Peter S. Uzelac, MD, FACOG
Assistant Professor
Department of Obstetrics and Gynecology
University of Southern California Keck School of Medicine
Los Angeles, California

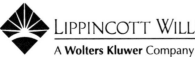 LIPPINCOTT WILLIAMS & WILKINS
A **Wolters Kluwer** Company
Philadelphia · Baltimore · New York · London
Buenos Aires · Hong Kong · Sydney · Tokyo

© 2005 by Michael A. Polisky, MD

351 West Camden Street
Baltimore, Maryland 21201-2436 USA

530 Walnut Street
Philadelphia, Pennsylvania 19106-3621 USA

The publisher is not responsible (as a matter of product liability, negligence, or otherwise) for any injury resulting from any material contained herein. This publication contains information relating to general principles of medical care which should not be construed as specific instructions for individual patients. Manufacturers' product information and package inserts should be reviewed for current information, including contraindications, dosages, and precautions.

ISBN: 978-1-4051-0434-0
ISBN: 1-4051-0434-1

Library of Congress Cataloging-in-Publication Data

Polisky, Michael A.
    SOAP for pediatrics / Michael A. Polisky, Breck Nichols.
        p. ; cm.
    Includes index.
    ISBN 1-4051-0434-1 (pbk.)
        1. Pediatrics—Handbooks, manuals, etc. 2. Children—Diseases—Handbooks, manuals, etc [DNLM: 1. Pediatrics—methods—Handbooks. WS 39 P768s 2005]
    I. Nichols, Breck. II. Title.

    RJ48.P65   2005
    618.92—dc22

                                                2004006157

A catalogue record for this title is available from the British Library

Editor: Donna Balado
Managing Editor: Kathleen Scogna
Marketing Manager: Emilie Linkins

The publishers have made very effort to trace the copyright holders for borrowed material. If they have inadvertently overlooked any, they will be pleased to make the necessary arrangements at the first opportunity.

To purchase additional copies of this book call our customer service department at (800) 638-3030 or fax orders to (301) 824-7390. International customers should call (301) 714-2324.

Visit Lippincott Williams & Wilkins on the Internet: http://www.lww.com. Lippincott Williams & Wilkins customer service representatives are available from 8:30 am to 6:00 pm, EST, Monday through Friday, for telephone access.

                                                4 5 6 7 8 9 10

To Keiko, you are my world. I could not have done this without you.

Paola, thank you for filling my life with happiness and love.

Thanks to our parents, patients, and professors for teaching us so much. We are truly standing on the shoulders of giants.

Contents

To the Reader

Like most medical students, I started my ward experience head down and running, eager to finally make contact with real patients. What I found was a confusing world, completely different from anything I had known during the first two years of medical school. New language, foreign abbreviations and residents too busy to set my bearings straight: Where would I begin?

Pocket textbooks, offering medical knowledge in a convenient and portable package, seemed to be the logical solution. Unfortunately, I found myself spending valuable time sifting through large amounts of text, often not finding the answer to my question, and in the process, missing out on teaching points during rounds!

I designed the SOAP series to provide medical students and house staff with pocket manuals that truly serve their intended purpose: quick accessibility to the most practical clinical information in a user-friendly format. At the inception of this project, I envisioned all of the benefits the SOAP format would bring to the reader:

- Learning through this model reinforces a thought process that is already familiar to students and residents, facilitating easier long-term retention.

- SOAP promotes good communication between physicians and facilitates the teaching/learning process.

- SOAP puts the emphasis back on the patient's clinical problem and not the diagnosis.

- In the age of managed care, SOAP meets the challenge of providing efficiency while maintaining quality.

- As sound medical-legal practice gains attention in physician training, SOAP emphasizes adherence to a documentation style that leaves little room for potential misinterpretation.

Rather than attempting to summarize the contents of a thousand-page textbook into a miniature form, the SOAP series focuses exclusively on guidance through patient encounters. In a typical use, "finding out where to start" or "refreshing your memory" with SOAP books should be possible in less than a minute. Subjects are always confined to two pages and the most important points have been highlighted. Topics have been limited to those problems you will most commonly encounter repeatedly during your training and contents are grouped according to the hospital or clinic setting. Facts and figures that are not particularly helpful to surviving life on the wards, such as demographics, pathophysiology and busy tables and graphs have purposely been omitted (such details are much better studied in a quiet environment using large and comprehensive texts).

Congratulations on your achievements thus far and I wish you a highly successful medical career!

Peter S. Uzelac, MD, FACOG

Acknowledgments

We wish to thank Drs. Lawrence Opas, Donna Elliot, Hrach Arutunyan, Craig Jones, Bernard Portnoy, Maureen McCollough, Jeff Johnson, Merujan Uzunyan, Cynthia Stotts, Carlos Luna, Frank Sinatra, Astrid Hegar, James Homans, Alvin Yusin, Robert Baehner, Susan McKenna, Rukmani Vasan, Linda Vachon, Jennifer Saenz, Rangasamy Ramanathan, Manuel Durand, Nancy Edwards, Diane Tanaka, Cecilia Essin, Y. Liza Kearl, Geetha Ramaswamy, Nabila Patel, Arno Hohn, Marc Weigensberg, and Laura Wachsman for all of their guidance and teaching.

A heartfelt debt of gratitude goes out to our parents and families for loving and supporting us.

Finally, we would like to thank Dr. Peter Uzelac for making this opportunity possible.

Reviewers

Kristy Anderson
Class of 2004
The University of Texas Health Science Center at San Antonio
San Antonio, Texas

Ayesha Bryant, MSPH
Class of 2005
University of Alabama School of Medicine
Birmingham, Alabama

Pamneit Bhogal
Class of 2005
Temple University School of Medicine
Philadelphia, Pennsylvania

David Gloss
Class of 2004
Tulane University School of Medicine
New Orleans, Louisiana

Abbreviations

AAP	American Academy of Pediatrics
ABC	airway breathing circulation
Abd	abdomen
ABG	arterial blood gas
ACE	angiotensin-converting enzyme
ADHD	attention deficit hyperactivity disorder
AFSFO	anterior fontanelle soft, flat, and open
AG	anion gap
AIDS	acquired immunodeficiency syndrome
ALT	alanine aminotransferase
ALTE	acute life-threatening event
AMS	altered mental status
ANA	antinuclear antibody
Anti-ENA-4	panel of rheumatologic labs
AP	anteroposterior
Appy	appendicitis
ARDS	acute respiratory distress syndrome
AS	aortic stenosis, auris sinister (left ear)
ASD	atrial septal defect
ASO	anti-streptolysin O titer
AST	aspartate aminotransferase
AV	atrioventricular
AVM	arteriovenous malformations
B	bilateral
Bicarb	bicarbonate
bid	*bis in die* (twice daily)
bili	bilirubin
BM	bowel movement, stool
BMI	body mass index
BS	bowel sounds
BSA	body surface area
BP	blood pressure
bpm	beats per minute
BUN	blood urea nitrogen
Ca	calcium
CAP	community-acquired pneumonia
CBC	complete blood count
cc	cubic centimeter
C/C/E	cyanosis/clubbing/edema
Chem 7	sodium, potassium, chloride, bicarb, BUN, creatinine, glucose
Chol	cholesterol
CK	creatinine kinase
CMV	cytomegalovirus
CN	cranial nerves
CNS	central nervous system
CP	chest pain
CPP	cerebral perfusion pressure

CPR	cardiopumonary resuscitation
Cr	creatinine
CRP	c-reactive protein
C-section	cesarean section
CSF	cerebrospinal fluid
CT	computed tomography, *Chlamydia trachomatis*
CTA	clear to auscultation
CV	cardiovascular
CVA	costovertebral angle, cerebrovascular accident
CXR	chest x-ray
D5$^1/_2$NS	5% dextrose in half normal saline
D10	a solution with 10% dextrose
D25	a solution with 25% dextrose
DBP	diastolic blood pressure
DIC	disseminated intravascular coagulation
Diff	differential
DKA	diabetic ketoacidosis
dL	deciliter
DM	diabetes mellitus
DTaP	Diphtheria, tetanus, and acellular pertussis vaccine
DTR	deep tendon reflexes
DVT	deep venous thrombosis
EBV	Epstein-Barr virus
ECG	electrocardiogram
EEG	electroencephalogram
ENT	ear, nose, and throat
EOMi	extraocular muscles intact
Epi	epinephrine
ER	emergency room
ESR	erythrocyte sedimentation rate
ETT	endotracheal tube
Ext	extremities
FB	foreign body
FEN	fluids electrolytes nutrition
FiO$_2$	fraction of inspired oxygen
g	gram
G6PD	glucose 6 phosphate dehydrogenase
GAS	group A streptoroccus
GBS	group B streptococcus
GC	gonococcus
GCS	Glasgow coma scale
Gen	general appearance of patient
GERD	gastroesophageal reflux disease
GI	gastrointestinal
Gluc	glucose
GTC	generalized tonic clonic
G-tube	gastrostomy tube
GU	genitourinary
H&P	history and physical
HBsAg	hepatitis B surface antigen

HBV	hepatitis B virus
HCO_3	bicarbonate
Hct	hematocrit
HEADSS	home, education, activities, drugs, sex, suicide
HEENT	head, eyes, ears, nose, throat
HELLP	hypertension, elevated liver enzymes, low platelets
Heme	hematologic
HIV	human immunodeficiency virus
HOCM	hypertrophic obstructive cardiomyopathy
HR	heart rate
hr	hour
HSP	Henoch-Schönlein purpura
HSV	herpes simplex virus
HUS	hemolytic uremic syndrome
Hz	Hertz
IBD	inflammatory bowel disease
IBS	irritable bowel syndrome
ICP	intracranial pressure
ICU	intensive care unit
ID	infectious disease
IDM	infant of diabetic mother
Ig	immunoglobulin
IM	intramuscular
IPV	inactivated poliovirus vaccine
ISAM	infant of a substance-abusing mother
ITP	idiopathic thrombocytopenic purpura
IV	intravenous
IVC	inferior vena cava
IVF	intravenous fluid
IVIG	intravenous immunoglobulin
JRA	juvenile rheumatoid arthritis
K	potassium
KD	Kawasaki disease
kg	kilogram
KUB	kidneys-ureter-bladder
L	left, liter
LAD	lymphadenopathy
Lat	lateral
LDH	lactate dehydrogenase
LFT	liver function test
LLQ	left lower quadrant
LOC	loss of consciousness
LP	lumbar puncture
LUQ	left upper quadrant
Lytes	electrolytes
MAP	mean arterial pressure
MCD	minimal change disease
mcg	microgram
MCP	metacarpophalangeal
MCV	mean cellular volume

mEq	milliequivalents
mg	milligram
Mg	magnesium
MI	myocardial infarction
min	minute
mL	milliliter
MMR	mumps, measles, rubella vaccine
Mono	mononucleosis
MPV	mean platelet volume
MRCP	mental retardation cerebral palsy
M/R/G/C	murmur/rub/gallop/click
MRI	magnetic resonance imaging
MV	minute ventilation
MVP	mitral valve prolapse
Na	sodium
NCAT	normocephalic atraumatic
ND	nondistended
NEC	necrotizing enterocolitis
Neuro	neurologic
NFEG	normal female external genitalia
NG	nasogastric
NICU	neonatal intensive care unit
NMEG	normal male external genitalia
NPH	neutral protamine Hagedorn insulin
NPO	*nulla per os* (nothing by mouth)
NRT	normal rectal tone
NS	normal saline
NSAID	nonsteroidal anti-inflammatory drug
NT	nontender
O_2	oxygen
O&P	ova and parasites
Ob/Gyn	obstetrics and gynecology
OP	oropharynx
OT	occupational therapy
P	pulse
PA	posteroanterior
PALS	pediatric advanced life support
PDA	patent ductus arteriosus
PE	physical exam
PEA	pulseless electrical activity
PEEP	positive end expiratory pressure
Perf'd Appy	perforated appendicitis
PERRLA	pupils equal, round, reactive to light, and accommodation
PGE_1	prostaglandin E_1
pH	negative log of the concentration of hydrogen
PICU	pediatric intensive care unit
PID	pelvic inflammatory disease
po	*per os* (by mouth)
Postop	postoperatively
PPD	purified protein derivative

preemie	premature baby
prn	*pro re nata* (as needed)
PS	pain score
pt	patient
PT	prothrombin time, physical therapy
PTT	partial thromboplastin time
Pulse ox	pulse oximeter
q	*quodque* (every)
qd	*quaque die* (once daily)
qh	*quaque hora* (every hour)
qhs	at bedtime
qid	*quater in die* (four times daily)
R	right, respirations
RBC	red blood cell
RDS	respiratory distress syndrome
Resp	respiratory
RF	rheumatic fever, rheumatoid factor
Rh	Rhesus factor
ROM	range of motion
RR	respiratory rate
RRR	regular rate and rhythm
RSV	respiratory syncytial virus
RLQ	right lower quadrant
RUQ	right upper quadrant
SBO	small bowel obstruction
SBP	systolic blood pressure
SCFE	slipped capital femoral epiphysis
Sec	seconds (time)
Ser	serum
SG	specific gravity
SH	Salter Harris
SLE	systemic lupus erythematosus
SM	systolic murmur
SQ	subcutaneous
STD	sexually transmitted disease
STI	sexually transmitted infection
SVC	superior vena cava
TB	tuberculosis
TBI	traumatic brain injury
TD	tetanus and diphtheria toxoids
tid	*ter in die* (three times daily)
TIG	tetanus immune globulin
TM	tympanic membrane
ToF	Tetralogy of Fallot
TSH	thyroid-stimulating hormone
TTN	transient tachypnea of the newborn
TTP	thrombotic thrombocytopenic purpura
U/A	urinalysis
UCx	urine culture
UOP	urine output

URI	upper respiratory infection
U/S	ultrasound
UTI	urinary tract infection
UV	ultraviolet
VCUG	vesiculocystourethrogram
V/Q	ventilation-perfusion
VSD	ventricular septal defect
WBC	white blood cell
WGA	weeks of gestational age
WPW	Wolff-Parkinson-White
wk	week
wt	weight

Normal Lab Values

Vitals. Approximate 95% confidence intervals. Means in parentheses where appropriate.

Age	Systolic BP	Diastolic BP	Heart Rate	Respiratory Rate
Term neonate	60–85 (70)	35–60 (55)	93–154 (123)	27–66 (43)
1 yr	70–100 (90)	40–60 (55)	89–151 (119)	20–49 (32)
2 yrs	72–105 (90)	40–60 (55)	89–151 (119)	17–39 (26)
3 yrs	74–110 (92)	40–65 (58)	73–137 (108)	16–34 (24)
5 yrs	78–112 (94)	45–70 (58)	65–133 (100)	16–31 (22)
8 yrs	86–117 (100)	45–75 (58)	62–130 (91)	16–24 (20)
12 yrs	94–125 (108)	50–80 (60)	60–119 (85)	14–23 (19)
>15 yrs	95–130 (115)	50–80 (60)	60–100 (72)	12–20 (16)

A fever is always T $\geq$ 100.4°F (38°C) rectally. Rectal can be up to 1°F higher than oral.

Hematology—Red blood cells and platelets.

Age	Hgb	Hct	MCV	Ferritin	Iron	ESR	Platelets
Preterm	13–15	42–47	118–120	—	—	—	254–290
Term	13.5–18.5	42–60	98–118	25–200	100–250	0–4	290
2 mos	9.4–13.0	28–42	84–106	50–200	40–100	—	252
6 mos–2 yrs	10.5–13.5	33–39	70–86	—	—	—	150–350
2 yrs–6 yrs	11.5–13.5	34–40	75–86	7–140	50–120	4–20	150–350
6 yrs–12 yrs	11.5–14.5	35–45	77–93	—	—	—	150–350
Adolescence							
male	13–15	36–50	78–98	7–140	65–175	0–10	150–350
female	12–14.5	37–45	78–98	7–140	50–170	0–20	150–350

Hematology—White blood cells and differential. CRP normal 0–0.5, all ages.

Age	WBC	% Neutrophils	% Lymphocytes	% Monocytes	% Eosinophils
Birth	9–30	55–87%	11–37%	6%	2%
12 hrs	13–38	64–74%	9–29%	5%	2%
24 hrs	9.4–34	55–81%	11–37%	6%	2%
2 wks	5–20	9–70%	18–85%	9%	3%
1 yr	6–17.5	32–49%	35–65%	5%	3%
4 yrs	5.5–15.5	37–50%	22–55%	5%	3%
6 yrs	5–14.5	42–60%	18–50%	5%	3%
10 yrs	4.5–13.5	45–65%	35–50%	4%	2%
>12 yrs	4.5–13	45–75%	30–45%	5%	3%

Serum Sodium (Na⁺)

Preterm	130–140 mEq/L
All others	136–145 mEq/L

Serum Potassium (K⁺)

<10 days old	4.0–6.0 mEq/L
>10 days old	3.5–5.1 mEq/L

Note: Children are notoriously difficult blood draws; hemolysis is a frequent complication and thus potassium is often falsely elevated.

Serum Chloride (Cl⁻)   99–111 mEq/L

Serum Bicarbonate (HCO₃⁻)

Preterm	18–26 mEq/L
Term	20–25 mEq/L
>2 yrs	22–26 mEq/L

Blood Urea Nitrogen (BUN)   7–22 mg/dL

Serum Creatinine (Cr)

Newborn	0.3–1.0 mg/dL
Infant	0.2–0.4 mg/dL
Child	0.3–0.7 mg/dL
Adolescent	Male: 0.6–1.3 mg/dL
	Female: 0.5–1.2 mg/dL

Serum Glucose

Preterm	45–100 mg/dL
Term	45–120 mg/dL
1 wk–16 yrs	60–105 mg/dL
>16 yrs	70–115 mg/dL

Serum Calcium (Ca⁺²)

Preterm	6–10 mg/dL
Full term	7–12 mg/dL
Child	8–10.5 mg/dL
Adolescent	8.5–10.5 mg/dL

Note: If albumin is low, calcium will be falsely depressed as well. The correction formula is: [4.0 - (serum albumin)](0.8) + [Ca⁺²].

Serum Magnesium (Mg⁺²)   1.7–2.2 mEq/dL

Serum Phosphorus (P)

Newborn	4.2–9.0 mg/dL
0–15 yrs	3.2–6.3 mg/dL
>15 yrs	2.7–4.5 mg/dL

Alkaline Phosphatase

Infant	150–420 U/L
2–10 yrs	100–320 U/L
11–18 yrs	Male: 100–390 U/L
	Female: 100–320 U/L

Albumin

Newborn	3.2–4.8 g/dL
1 mo	2.5–5.5 g/dL
3 mos	2.1–4.8 g/dL
6 mos	2.8–5.0 g/dL
1 yr	3.2–5.7 g/dL
2 yrs	1.9–5.0 g/dL
3 yrs	3.3–5.8 g/dL
5 yrs	2.9–5.8 g/dL
8 yrs	3.2–5.0 g/dL
>16 yrs	3.1–5.4 g/dL

Bilirubin (Total)

Age	Preterm	Term
0–1 day	<8 mg/dL	<6 mg/dL
1–2 days	<12 mg/dL	<8 mg/dL
3–5 days	<16 mg/dL	<12 mg/dL
After	0.1–1.2 mg/dL	

Direct or Conjugated Bilirubin should always be <0.4 mg/dL.

Aspartate Aminotransferase (AST/SGOT)

Infant	20–65 U/L
Child/Adolescent	0–35 U/L

Alanine Aminotransferase (ALT/SGPT)

Infant	<54 U/L
Child/adolescent	1–60 U/L

Creatine Kinase (CK/CPK)

Newborn	10–200 U/L
All others	Male: 12–80 U/L
	Female: 10–55 U/L

Lactate Dehydrogenase (LD/LDH)

Neonate	160–1500 U/L
Infant	150–360 U/L
Child	150–300 U/L
Adolescent	0–220 U/L

Lipids. HDL should always be >45 mg/dL.

	Desirable	Borderline	High
Total Cholesterol (mg/dL)	<170	170–199	≥200
Low Density Lipoprotein (mg/dL)	<110	110–129	≥160

Lead. Normal lead is 0!

Acceptable serum lead level   <10 mcg/dL

Osmolality   285–295 mOsm/kg

Fibrinogen   200–400 mg/dL

Antinuclear Antibody (ANA)

<1:80   Not significant

>1:320   Significant

Rheumatoid factor   <20 conventional units

Sex Hormones

	LH (mIU/mL)	FSH (mIU/mL)	Testosterone (ng/dL)	Estradiol (pg/mL)
Prepubertal children	0–1.6	0–2.8	10–20	<25
Postpubertal				
Male	1–10.2	1.4–14.4	275–875	6–44
Female			23–75	
Luteal				15–260
Follicular	0.9–14	3.7–12.9		10–200
Midcycle				120–375
Pregnant			35–195	

Serum Cortisol

Pre-ACTH in AM	5.7–16.6
1 hour post-ACTH	16–36

Diabetic labs

Insulin (fasting)	1.8–24.6 mcU/mL
C-peptide (fasting)	0.8–4.0 ng/mL
Hemoglobin A1C	4.5–6.1%

Thyroid Function Tests

Age	T_4 (mcg/dL)	T_3 (ng/dL)	TSH (mIU/mL)	TBG (mg/dL)
1–3 days	11.0–21.5	100–380	<2.5–13.3	0.7–4.7
1–4 wks	8.2–16.6	99–310	0.6–10.0	0.5–4.5
1–12 mos	7.2–15.6	102–264	0.6–6.3	1.6–3.6
1–5 yrs	7.3–15.0	105–269	" "	1.3–2.8
6–10 yrs	6.4–13.3	94–241	" "	1.4–2.6
11–15 yrs	5.6–11.7	83–213	" "	" "
≥16 yrs	4.2–11.8	80–210	0.2–7.6	" "

I

Newborn Nursery

S Obtain a maternal social Hx.

Important for determining safety of the neonate.
- Maternal sexually transmitted infections (STIs: GC, CT, HSV, syphilis, HBV, HIV)
- Mother's occupation
- Previous children
- Maternal illicit drug use
- Where the baby will live

Has the mother had prenatal care and labs? Has she been taking any medications?

Between the mother and her chart, record whether she has the following risk factors:
- Urine culture positive for Group B strep   - HIV
- Diabetes mellitus   - Hepatitis
- TB

Medications that can have an adverse effect on the baby include:
- Antiepileptics   - Narcotics
- Antibiotics   - Antihypertensives

O Examine the baby under a radiant warmer. Review vital signs. Additions to a general physical exam include:

Measurements: Length, weight, and head circumference

Head: Palpate scalp, anterior and posterior fontanelle; check to make sure the sutures move.

Eyes: Look for a red reflex with an ophthalmoscope.

Palate: Check for cleft (sometimes a finger may need to be inserted into the mouth for this).

Ears: Look for tags, and make sure the superior attachment is level with the eye. If it is not, we say the ears are low-set, a possible sign of a genetic disorder.

Hands and feet: Look for extra digits.

Musculoskeletal: Look for clavicular fractures, sacral spine for pits, dimples, or hair tufts.

Abdomen: Palpate both kidneys. Unusual masses should also be palpable.

Pulses: Place one finger on a femoral pulse and the other on the right brachial pulse. They should be equal and occur at the same time, without delay.

Hips: Perform Ortolani (**O**ut) and Barlow (**B**ack) maneuvers (feeling for clunks).
- Ortolani maneuver is performed by grasping the proximal thighs with the index finger on the greater trochanter and the thumb on the lesser trochanter and abducting the hips 180 degrees. If a clunk is felt, you have reduced a dislocated hip.
- Barlow maneuver is performed by using the same grasp on adducted hips and pushing down toward the table. If a clunk is felt, you have dislocated the hip.

Infant neuro exam:
- *Moro:* Support the head and make the baby feel as if s/he is falling back. The arms should go out symmetrically, fingers splayed, with a small shake.
- *Gallant:* Place the baby face down in the palm of your hand, stroke back on L or R, baby's bottom moves to side stroked.
- Palmar and plantar grasp, baby's tone, suck, jitteriness, and for tolerance of feeds.

Skin: Look for any normal or abnormal lesions or jaundice (see Benign Skin Lesions p. 6 and Jaundice p. 24).

Ballard exam (a neurologic and physical maturity scale) is used to estimate gestational age.

A **Normal Newborn: Decide if the neonate requires a workup for sepsis.**
Maternal characteristics to suggest an amnionitis workup:
- Membranes ruptured   - Group B strep (+)   - Uterine tenderness
  >18 hours   - Fever at delivery
- Foul-smelling lochia

Neonatal characteristics to suggest an amnionitis workup:
- <37 wks' gestation   - Fetal tachycardia   - Grunting

The amnionitis workup consists of a CBC with differential, CRP, and blood culture. If results are abnormal, transfer the baby to the neonatal intensive care unit (NICU) for presumed sepsis.

Consider transfer to the NICU if:
Baby's weight is less than 2250 g or more than 4500 g.
Mother is diabetic using insulin or had a sugar over 120.
Gestational age of the baby by Ballard or dates is less than 35 wks.
Baby has symptoms of distress:
- Accessory respiratory muscle use   - Grunting
- Nasal flaring   - Cyanosis

P **Consider all things that may endanger the neonate before discharge at 48 to 72 hrs.**
Rule out subgaleal hemorrhage. Follow CBCs and vital signs if suspected.
Subgaleal hemorrhage: If scalp bogginess extends to the back of the neck, observe carefully because a baby can lose its entire blood volume into this space.

For an abnormal red reflex, refer to ophthalmology:
Red reflex abnormalities can mean cataracts, strabismus, or retinoblastoma.

Order an echocardiogram if the cardiovascular exam is abnormal.
Murmurs may be congenital heart lesions. Pulse differentials can be a coarcted aorta.

If the hip exam is abnormal, refer for U/S of the hips and then to orthopedics.
Hip clunks on the Ortolani and Barlow can be signs of developmental dysplasia of the hip. If the problem is not corrected in early infancy, the child may never walk.

For an abnormal infant neuro exam, consult a pediatric neurologist.
Also, if the exam is asymmetric, consider birth trauma, such as a brachial plexus injury.

Check a total bilirubin on the second day of life. Consider NICU transfer if >10.
A neonate sent home with a rapidly climbing bilirubin is at risk for kernicterus.

Explain normal and abnormal skin findings to the parents.
See Benign Skin Lesions p. 6.

Use the Ballard exam estimate for gestational age only if it is more than 2 wks different from the prebirth estimated gestational age.
This is a predetermined pediatric scale.

Vaccinate for hepatitis B. If mom is HBsAg (+) or status is unknown, give HBV IgG.

S **Were there any complications in the delivery?**
Trauma risks include:
- Breech presentation   - Vacuum extraction   - Forceps extraction
- Scalp electrode   - Cesarean section (scalpel lacerations)

What are the physical characteristics of the mother?
Trauma risks include:
- Primiparity →   - Small vaginal canal contractions - Strong uterine
- Maternal short stature - Pelvic anomalies

How long was the labor?
Prolonged or rapid labor may also be risk factors to the neonate.

What are the physical characteristics of the neonate or amniotic sac?
Oligohydramnios (less than normal amount of amniotic fluid surrounding the baby)
increases risk of trauma to baby because of less fluid protecting it from the initial
uterine contractions.
A baby with a large head (e.g., hydrocephalus) or shoulders (e.g., macrosomic) may
have difficulty passing through the birth canal.

O **Trauma is most commonly seen in the following areas:**
Head (the largest and most common presenting part of the fetus)
Caput succedaneum (most common and benign type of extracranial hemorrhage):
Occurs when serosanguineous fluid collects in the subcutaneous area between the
galea aponeurotica and the skin. It is boggy in texture with poorly defined margins
and crosses suture lines.
Cephalohematoma: A subperiosteal collection of blood caused by rupture of a blood
vessel on the surface of the bone presenting as a firm, discrete mass that does not cross
suture lines. Underlying skull fracture is sometimes present. Rarely associated with
significant hemorrhage.
Subgaleal hemorrhage (most dangerous and least common extracranial hemorrhage):
Caused by bleeding between the periosteum and the galea aponeurotica. It is a large
space, extending from the orbital ridge over the entire skull to the ears and back of the
neck, into which the neonate's entire blood volume can be lost. Examine carefully for
bogginess, fluctuance, or pitting edema in this entire region.

Exam of the neck and shoulders
Torticollis: The head is held tilted to one side with a palpable sternocleidomastoid mass
possibly resulting from birth trauma or intrauterine positioning.
Clavicular fracture (most common neonatal orthopedic injury): Crepitus
(crunchy/crackling) or bony irregularity along the clavicle. Often occurs during
delivery of the shoulders or shoulder dystocia.

Exam of the arms
Erb's palsy: Injury of the fifth and sixth cervical spinal roots, causing the arm to be
adducted, internally rotated, with the elbow extended, forearm prone, and wrist
flexed. Because the fingers are not involved, palmar grasp reflex is present, but Moro is
absent.
Klumpke's palsy (rare): Traction of the seventh and eighth cervical nerves, and first
thoracic nerve, causing flexed elbow, supinated forearm, extended wrist, and
hyperextension of the MCP joints. Grasp is absent. Moro is present.
Entire plexus injury causes an entirely flaccid arm.

Exam of the skin

Petechiae (common): Nonblanching red spots caused by subcutaneous capillary bleeding

Ecchymosis (bruise): Larger nonblanching areas of subcutaneous bleeding

Lacerations (common): Cuts in the skin from scalpels, forceps, or other trauma

Subcutaneous fat necrosis (usually occurs a day or two after birth): Presents as irregularly shaped reddish purple subcutaneous nodules, which are hard to the touch. Often resulting from instrumentation, such as forceps, on the cheek of the baby.

Sucking blisters: Bullae or ulcerations on the wrist, finger, foot, etc. caused by sucking in utero

A **Birth trauma. A small DDx includes:**

Excessive petechiae or subcutaneous bleeding should be ruled out for sepsis and bleeding diathesis such as hemophilia or platelet disorders.

Extensive fractures should be ruled out for osteogenesis imperfecta or other bone disorders.

Mongolian spots (see Benign Skin Lesions p. 6) can be mistaken for ecchymoses.

P **Always keep the parents well-informed.**

This will prevent panic if they find trauma incidentally.

Note and record all injuries in the chart.

This should prevent legal action against the obstetrician or pediatrician.

For caput succedaneum and cephalohematoma, confirm that they are not evolving subgaleal hemorrhages. Check CBCs and T bili levels. Take a skull x-ray if skull fracture is suspected.

Blood breakdown in these injuries can elevate total bilirubin and lead to jaundice.

If subgaleal hemorrhage is suspected, monitor for signs of volume loss, such as tachycardia and hypotension. Check CBCs. Replace blood and fluids as needed.

This should be sufficient to prevent hypovolemic shock in these high-risk neonates.

For torticollis, observe, massage, perform gentle stretching, and place a pillow on the affected side to hold the head away from the shoulders while sleeping.

This therapy has been shown to correct torticollis in a matter of weeks to months.

If clavicular fractures are suspected, perform an x-ray to confirm the diagnosis.

Nothing else needs to be done except to follow up with x-rays to verify callus formation and normal healing.

For brachial plexus injuries, nothing needs to be done.

These usually resolve in 1 to 2 wks. The pt should have neurologic follow-up. No improvement by 6 months indicates a poor prognosis.

Suture all wide or deep lacerations.

S **Are there any genetic disorders in the family that may present with skin lesions?**

Neurofibromatosis (von Recklinghausen disease): Can present with multiple, large café-au-lait spots, axillary freckling. In the neonate, more than three spots or any one spot larger than 3 cm should make you suspicious for this disease.

Tuberous sclerosis: Multiple fibromas, ash-leaf spots, Shagreen patch, Lisch nodules

Waardenburg syndrome: Presents with piebaldism, partial areas of hypopigmentation.

Peutz-Jeghers syndrome: Presents in the neonatal period with multiple, scattered hyperpigmented macules usually found on the nose, mouth, fingers, hands, and mucous membranes of the mouth. Usually associated with intestinal polyps.

Albright's syndrome: In adults, it has bony lesions and endocrine abnormalities. In neonates, it presents with a single, large (up to 12 cm), ragged, irregular hyperpigmented lesion.

O **Lesions can be red, brown, white, or blue and can be raised or flat**

Raised red lesions:

Erythema toxicum: One of the most common findings on the skin of the neonate. It usually looks like small red marks on the skin, with tiny papules arising from the center of each red macule. It can occur anywhere on the body. It is far more common in healthy, term neonates.

Staphylococcal skin infections: Be sure to differentiate them from erythema toxicum. The pustules are usually grouped periumbilically, in the axillae, or groin.

Superficial hemangioma: The old term for this kind of lesion is strawberry hemangioma, and this is highly descriptive. It would be rare in the nursery to have a fully recognizable strawberry hemangioma, but, if present, it would appear as a raised, red nodule, or it may appear as a pale macule with some blood vessels appearing within it.

Flat red lesions:

Nevus simplex (salmon patch, stork bite): Usually pink, not red. It is approximately $^1/_2$ to 1 cm in size. The most common location is on the nape of the neck, but it may also be found on the forehead, eyelid, or bridge of the nose. It is extremely common.

Port-wine stain (nevus flammeus): Usually unilateral, reddish-purple, and commonly found on the face. If it involves the area of the ophthalmic branch of the trigeminal nerve, this is known as Sturge-Weber syndrome.

Raised brown lesions:

Nevi: These form when groups of melanocytes are grouped together. Junctional nevi are small and benign. Compound nevi are similar, but they may be hairy and slightly larger. The most obvious is the giant hairy nevus, which may cover 20% to 30% of the total body surface area.

Flat brown lesions:

Transient pustular melanosis: Difficult to categorize because it may have red raised lesions and brown flat lesions at both extremes. More common in African-American babies. Noninfectious pustules rupture to form raised, then flat brown spots on the skin, then resolve.

Raised blue lesions:

Deep hemangioma: The new term for cavernous hemangioma. Like superficial hemangioma, this is a vascular malformation. It is deep in the skin but tends to cause a raised blue lesion. If it is large, it can sequester blood and platelets (Kasabach-Merritt syndrome).

Flat blue lesions:
Mongolian spots: More common in babies of African or Asian descent. Usually disappear by the age of 3 years. Tend to appear blue, like bruising. They can be small or large and occur anywhere, although the lumbosacral region is most common. It is important to note them because they fade slowly and later may make someone suspicious for child abuse.

Raised white lesions:
Milia (common): Epidermal cysts appear as tiny white papules on the nose, forehead, and chin.
Sebaceous gland hyperplasia: Like milia, but the papules are smaller and grouped together.

Flat white lesions:
Piebaldism and ash-leaf spots as noted above are the main hypopigmented lesions.

It is important to note that there is also a lesion of absent skin:
Cutis aplasia: Occurs when the skin does not form. This usually occurs over the midline of the posterior scalp. It looks like a punched-out area (with no hair) 1 to 2 cm in diameter.

Often you will find more than one lesion in the same pt.

Benign skin lesions. DDx includes:
Child abuse: Consider in the case of Mongolian spots and cutis aplasia. However, it is unlikely to occur in the hospital.
Heat rash: May appear similar to erythema toxicum.

All of these lesions are initially benign. Some may require later intervention.

Lesions that require no intervention and will self-resolve:
- Transient neonatal pustular melanosis
- Nevus simplex
- Sebaceous gland hyperplasia
- Small deep hemangioma
- Erythema toxicum
- Junctional nevi
- Superficial hemangioma
- Mongolian spots
- Milia

Giant hairy nevi and compound nevi have the potential to become malignant in the future and should be surgically removed.
Refer to surgery or dermatology clinic.

Port-wine stains are cosmetically undesirable and require pulse-dye laser therapy. Obtain an MRI of the brain for suspected Sturge-Weber pts.
An MRI is needed because Sturge-Webber pts can have underlying brain lesions.

Large deep hemangiomas may require surgical resection.
If large enough, they can cause anemia, thrombocytopenia, and high-output heart failure.

Place a surgical dressing over cutis aplasia.
This will prevent injury or infection.

II

Neonatal Intensive Care Unit

S **Did the mother have prenatal care?**
A history of prenatal care decreases the risk of postbirth complications.

Does the mother have signs of infection?
- Membranes ruptured   - Group B strep (+)   - Uterine tenderness
  > 18 hrs   - Fever at delivery
- Foul-smelling lochia

Does the mother have any chronic illnesses that may increase the risk of complications?
- Diabetes mellitus   - Hypertension   - Lupus
- Hypothyroidism   - Hyperthyroidism

Is there a history of problems with previous deliveries?
A history of problems may help you prepare for one today.

Is the mother taking any medications or did she receive any during delivery?
Medications that can have an adverse effect on the baby include:
- Antiepileptics   - Narcotics   - Antibiotics
- Antihypertensives   - Magnesium

Does the mother have pregnancy-related problems such as pregnancy-induced hypertension; hypertension, elevated liver enzymes, low platelets (HELLP syndrome); or gestational diabetes?
As noted above, hypertension and diabetes increase the risk of complications.

Are there any signs of distress in the baby, such as tachycardia or decelerations?
These signs may indicate a more difficult resuscitation.

What is the estimated gestational age and weight of the baby?
Infants less than 35 wks or 2250 g are more likely to have respiratory difficulty at birth.

O **Set up for delivery.**
Turn on the radiant warmer, the O_2, and the suction. Attach the suction catheter.

Get supplies.
Warm towels, blankets, cap, and a cord clamp
Intubation supplies (laryngoscope with 0 and 1 blades; 2.5 [1000 g neonates], 3.0 [1000–2000 g], 3.5 [2000–3000 g], and 4.0 [>3000 g] endotracheal tubes [ETTs], and stylet).
  • Check to make sure the light on the blade of the laryngoscope turns on and that it is firmly attached (but don't leave it on because it becomes very hot).

Receiving the baby
Position, suction, dry, and stimulate (by drying off back with warm towel).
Change out towels after 1 to 2 minutes, as they become wet.

Table I APGAR Scores			
	0	1	2
Appearance	Blue	Blue hands and feet	Pink
Pulse	Absent	<100	>100
Grimace	None	Grimace	Cough/sneeze/crying
Activity	No tone	Slightly flexed	Moves all extremities
Respirations	Absent	Slow	Crying

Perform APGARs at 1 and 5 minutes and then every 5 minutes after that until an APGAR over 7 is achieved (see Table 1).

Examine the lungs for clear breath sounds. Repeat suctioning if rales are present.

 Newborn baby in active resuscitation. Assess the APGAR scores.
A good order for the APGARs is HRTIC. Heart rate is the most important: the last you will lose, and the first you will get back. If this score is 1 or less, you need to know that immediately. Color is the first sign you will lose and the last you will get back. APGAR scores tell you little about prognosis; only whether to continue the resuscitation.

Remember that if the mother has lupus, this may cause congenital third-degree heart block. Consider this if you are unable to raise the heart rate with conventional CPR.

The differential of low APGAR scores is as follows (GOVAKS TIPS MD):

- Glucose (hypoglycemia)
- O_2 (hypoxia)
- Volume (hypovolemia)
- Acidosis (consider giving Bicarb)
- K (hypo/hyperkalemia)
- Seizure (hypoCa/gluc)
- Temp (hypothermia, fever)
- Internal Bleed (subgaleal)
- Pneumothorax (bag-valve-mask)
- Surfactant (ROS p. 114)
- Meconium (suction well)
- Drugs (consider Narcan)

P **If the APGAR is ≤7, then continue down this path until you achieve that score:**
1. Blow by oxygen × 30 sec –>
2. Bag-valve-mask gently (avoid causing a pneumothorax), look for adequate chest rise –>
3. CPR (two fingers just below nipple line) –>
4. Intubate (usually 0 blade, 3.0 ETT) –>
5. Umbilical vein line (using a 3.5 or 5 Fr catheter, insert 1 to 4 cm at point where good blood return occurs) –>
6. Normal saline bolus 10 cc/kg up to 3 times and then consider transfusion –>
7. Epinephrine 0.01 mL/kg –>
8. Narcan 0.1 mg/kg –>
9. Dopamine 5 mcg/kg/min titrate to a normal BP/mean arterial pressure

If congenital third-degree heart block is suspected, start emergent transcutaneous pacing.

Decide if the neonate requires a workup for sepsis (CBC, CRP, and blood culture).

Maternal characteristics to suggest an amnionitis workup:
- Membranes ruptured   - Group B strep (+)   - Uterine tenderness
  >18 hours   - Fever at delivery
- Foul-smelling lochia

Neonatal characteristics to suggest an amnionitis workup:
- <37 wks' gestation   - Fetal tachycardia   - Grunting

Consider admission to NICU if:
Baby's weight is less than 2250 g or more than 4500 g.
Mother is a diabetic using insulin or had a sugar over 120.
Gestational age of the baby is less than 35 wks.
Baby has any symptoms of distress, such as grunting, nasal flaring, use of accessory muscles of respiration, or cyanosis.

All of the other babies (the majority of them) will be normal and go to the newborn nursery.

S **Is your pt premature?**

Transient tachypnea of the newborn (TTN) is a diagnosis of exclusion. It is generally a mild form of respiratory distress. It rarely occurs in premature babies; in these pts, respiratory difficulty is more likely to be premature lung disease or respiratory distress syndrome (RDS).

How long did labor last?

The greatest risk factor for TTN is a lack of labor. During labor, uterine contractions stimulate increased lymphatic uptake. TTN occurs because there is a failure to take up lymphatic fluid from the lungs.

Was there a delay in clamping the cord?

If the pt receives a postnatal transfusion from the placenta, resulting in an increased circulating blood volume, this is also a risk factor for increased lymphatic fluid in the lungs.

Are any other factors present associated with increased risk?

Male sex and fetal macrosomia

Are there any maternal risk factors for sepsis?

TTN must be differentiated from pneumonia, which can be a presentation of sepsis. See Rule Out Sepsis/Meningitis (p. 26) for a complete discussion of the risks.

O **How long has it been since delivery?**

TTN can present during the resuscitation. However, neonates with respiratory distress during resuscitation likely have other problems. TTN usually presents 2 to 6 hrs after delivery.

What are the pt's clinical symptoms?

Tachypnea is the hallmark feature. Respiratory rate will usually be greater than 80. The neonate will also likely display other signs of respiratory distress. These include:

- *Grunting:* A coarse, guttural sound made with each expiration. This is an effort to increase the end expiratory pressure by exhaling against a closed glottis (vocal cords), which helps the baby keep the alveoli open.
- *Retractions:* In an effort to counter decreased pulmonary compliance, the neonate may pull with the intercostal and subcostal muscles, a sign of distress.
- *Nasal flaring:* Also a sign of respiratory distress.

Presence of tachypnea without other signs of respiratory distress may indicate central hyperventilation, as in infants with birth asphyxia. An arterial blood gas will show respiratory alkalosis.

The neonate may appear mildly cyanotic.

Does the pt have any findings on auscultation of the lungs?

Lungs should sound clear with good air exchange. There should be no crackles or rhonchi.

How much oxygen is required to maintain a peripheral O_2 saturation greater than 90%?

A fraction of inspired oxygen (FiO_2) is usually less than 40%. If the newborn requires 60% or more, or mechanical ventilation, consider another diagnosis, such as RDS, rather than TTN.

Obtain a chest x-ray.
Radiograph of the chest in TTN will usually show prominent perihilar streaking.
Fluid in the minor fissure (a horizontal line across the right lung on AP chest x-ray) or small pleural fluid are also common.
Coarse, fluffy densities in the lungs caused by fluid-filled alveoli usually resolve in <24 hrs.
Increased lung volume (flattened diaphragms) occurs secondary to air trapping.

Obtain a CBC, CRP, and blood culture.
Indicators of sepsis should be normal. The WBC count should not be excessively low (less than 5), and there should not be a bandemia. The CRP should remain less than 3.0, and a blood culture should remain negative. Otherwise, treat your pt as if septic.

Perform a hyperoxia test (see Cyanosis p. 18).
A positive hyperoxia test should make you think of congenital heart lesions as an etiology.

A **Transient Tachypnea of the Newborn**
TTN (type II RDS) occurs when resorption of fetal lung fluid by the pulmonary lymphatic system is delayed. This fluid sits in the peribronchial lymphatics waiting to be reabsorbed. The increased fluid exerts pressure on the bronchi, causing them to close off. Thus air is trapped in the lungs via a mechanism similar to asthma. As with asthma, hypoxia occurs when blood circulates through alveoli that are poorly ventilated, thus creating a ventilation-perfusion (commonly known as V/Q) mismatch. The excess fluid makes the lungs less compliant, and the neonate breathes faster and develops retractions to compensate.

Differential diagnosis:
- Sepsis   - Pneumonia   - Premature
- Central hyperventilation   - Congenital heart lesions   lung disease

P **Support your pt through this illness.**
Remember the diagnosis: *transient* tachypnea of the newborn. This will go away on its own.

Place the pt in an oxyhood or on a nasal cannula if hypoxic.
This should support the neonate until the fluid is reabsorbed.

Consider providing nasal continuous positive airway pressure to help maintain the bronchi open if hypoxia persists at an FiO$_2$ of 40%. Feed orally or via an orogastric tube.
IV fluid should not be necessary in most cases.

Symptoms and x-ray findings should resolve in 48 to 72 hrs.

S **What is the baby's gestational age?**
Surfactant is not at mature levels in the right areas until after 32 wks' gestation. The lower the gestational age, the higher the risk of neonatal respiratory distress syndrome (RDS), also called hyaline membrane disease.

Does the pt have any risk factors for RDS?

- Delivery <37 wks   - Elective C-section   - Multiple gestation
- Maternal diabetes   - Birth asphyxia   - Intubation
- Cold stress   - Siblings with RDS

- During labor, steroid and adrenergic production in the mother stimulate fetal surfactant release. Therefore, delivery without a trial of labor (elective c-section) increases the risk of RDS.
- Birth asphyxia, pneumonia, aspiration, oxygen toxicity, barotrauma, or volutrauma can all lead to deficiencies of surfactant, which can cause or exacerbate RDS.

Are there any factors that may decrease the risk of RDS?

- Pregnancy-induced hypertension   - Antenatal corticosteroids
- Opiate addiction   - Prolonged rupture of membranes
- The best way to treat RDS is to prevent it before it occurs. If it is known in advance that the delivery will be premature, the mother should receive dexamethasone or betamethasone more than 24 hrs and less than 7 days beforehand. If possible, an earlier dose of corticosteroids given 1 wk before delivery has also been shown to be beneficial.

O **Look for symptoms of respiratory distress.**

- Tachypnea   - Shallow respirations   - Grunting
- Cyanosis   - Intercostal retractions   - Subcostal retractions
- Nasal flaring

- These symptoms should occur within minutes of birth. If the symptoms occur several hours later, then they have not been noted or there is an alternative diagnosis, such as sepsis, aspiration of feeds, or closure of a patent ductus arteriosus in a ductal dependent heart lesion.
- If there is cyanosis out of proportion to the respiratory distress or a heart murmur, consider the possibility of a congenital heart malformation.

Obtain a chest x-ray.
Usually, the chest x-ray will have a ground glass appearance that is typical but not pathognomonic for RDS. Note that the chest x-ray may appear normal until even as late as 12 hrs of life.
Other abnormalities that may be seen include an abnormally shaped heart, pneumothorax, pneumomediastinum, pleural effusion, diaphragmatic hernia, and meconium aspiration. All of these will show up with characteristic findings on the chest x-ray.

Check an ABG, CBC, CRP, and blood culture.
The ABG will help decide how aggressive respiratory intervention needs to be and can give some clues about possible comorbid or alternative diagnoses.
CBC, CRP, and blood culture can help assess both the possibility of infection as well as anemia or polycythemia.

A **Neonatal Respiratory Distress Syndrome**
RDS occurs when the neonate fails to make sufficient surfactant to coat the insides of the alveoli. Surfactant is a combination of protein and phospholipids that reduces the surface tension of water in the lungs, allowing the alveoli to remain patent and preventing collapse.

Differential diagnosis/comorbidities
Infection
  • Group B strep (mimicking or coexisting with RDS)
Congenital heart malformation
  • Total anomalous pulmonary venous return
  • Transposition of the great vessels
  • Hypoplastic left heart
Aspiration
  • Meconium (may cause secondary surfactant inactivation).
  • Feeds (indicates possible tracheoesophageal fistula or neurologic deficit).
Transient tachypnea of the newborn: Self-resolves in 24 to 48 hrs.

P **Provide respiratory support as needed to keep oxygen saturations >90%. Begin with supplemental O$_2$ by oxyhood, and escalating to continous positive airway pressure via nasal prongs, then intubation on conventional or even high-frequency ventilation if necessary.**
The difficulty with ventilating these pts is finding a way, if at all possible, to maintain sats without delivering a toxic level of oxygen, or using too much or too little pressure.
  • If pressure is too high while ventilating, pt may develop a pneumothorax.
  • If pressure is too low, further damage may result as the alveoli collapse and reexpand with each breath.

Give a dose of surfactant directly down the endotracheal tube.
A dose of surfactant shortly after birth helps reduce the mortality but not morbidity of RDS. Multidose therapy can also be used if the baby is intubated and requires an FiO$_2$ > 30%.

S **Were there any risk factors for meconium passage?**
Late delivery or being postdates
  • In one study, more than 30% of all pregnancies that lasted longer than 42 wks
    had passage of meconium.
These other causes of uteroplacental insufficiency are also a risk for meconium passage:
          - Uterine infection   - Maternal sepsis   - Hypertension
          - Smoking   - Long-standing diabetes   - Heart disease
          - Chronic lung disease

Was meconium visualized on delivery of the neonate or on rupture of the amnion?
Meconium aspiration can occur with minimal meconium, but it is more common
  when there is more of it in the amniotic fluid.

What was the appearance of the meconium?
Meconium in the amnion that has been there for a while may appear yellow, thin, and
  watery. This is possibly less risky than the thick, particulate, pea soup–appearing,
  fresh meconium.

Was an effort made to remove meconium from the pt's airway before the first breath?
During the resuscitation of a neonate bathed in meconium, particularly thick
  meconium, suctioning of the mouth and nares is generally not sufficient. The larynx
  should have been directly visualized to search for meconium, and an endotracheal
  tube inserted in order to act as a meconium suction catheter. This should be done
  before the neonate makes its first respiratory efforts in order to prevent meconium
  particles from passing deep into the lungs. If this is done, the risk of aspiration is less.
  However, this is not definite as aspiration often occurs before birth.

O **Look for physical signs of meconium staining.**
Meconium that has just been passed will not have stained the neonate. Long-standing
  meconium will turn the neonate's umbilical cord and finger and toenails yellow/green.

What is the current respiratory status of the neonate?
Not all infants who aspirate meconium do poorly. In fact, two-thirds of all neonates
  who have been suctioned in the delivery room will be asymptomatic, even with an
  abnormal chest x-ray (CXR).
Signs of respiratory distress include:
          - Tachypnea   - Shallow respirations   - Grunting
          - Cyanosis   - Intercostal retractions   - Subcostal retractions
          - Nasal flaring
Auscultate the chest for rales and rhonchi, which may be present.

Check O_2 sat and an arterial blood gas.
The clearest signs of respiratory distress are hypoxia (low O_2 sat, low pO_2) and
  hypercapnia (high pCO_2).

Send blood for a CBC with differential, a CRP, and a culture.
Pts with meconium aspiration require a septic workup (see Rule Out Sepsis/Meningitis
  p. 26).

Check a CXR.
Aspirated meconium appears as blotchy infiltrates in both lungs.

Meconium aspiration
Meconium is the neonate's first stool passage. Ordinarily and physiologically, it does not occur until after birth. When it occurs before birth, there is a risk of aspirating it into the lungs. It is thick, sticky, and black-green in color. Unlike later stools, it is not infiltrated with bacteria.

Meconium is passed when the fetus is either acutely or chronically hypoxic. The hypoxia stimulates not only meconium passage but also gasping, increasing the chances that meconium floating in the amnion will find its way into the lungs. You may imagine that having a thick, sticky material in the parenchyma of the lungs is not good. It can cause various problems (e.g., mechanical obstruction, chemical pneumonitis, inactivation of surfactant), all of which make it difficult to oxygenate and ventilate the pt.

This causes a problem similar to that seen in premature lung disease. When the airway is obstructed, the alveoli may collapse (atelectasis). When blood runs through collapsed alveoli, it receives no oxygen. This is known as a ventilation-perfusion (V/Q) mismatch, and it is responsible for most hypoxia.

The pt is also at risk for pneumothorax, pneumomediastinum, and pulmonary hypertension.

Differential diagnosis:
Congenital heart disease
Diaphragmatic hernia
Pneumonia
Central hyperventilation
Hypoplastic lungs
Sepsis
  • Sepsis should be ruled out regardless because meconium aspiration is a sign of distress in utero, and amnionitis is one of the leading causes of distress.

P **Support the pt's ventilatory efforts. Give oxygen by oxyhood or nasal cannula for hypoxia. If the problem persists, the pt may be placed on nasal continuous positive airway pressure.**
This will force open the airways that are obstructed, decrease the atelectasis, and decrease the V/Q mismatch.

Consider intubation and mechanical ventilation for rising pCO_2. High-frequency oscillatory ventilation may be more effective than conventional ventilation because it allows for efficient ventilation at lower volumes.
High-volume ventilation is problematic because of the plugging of the airways, atelectasis, inactivation of surfactant, and air trapping caused by the sticky meconium.

Consider giving a dose of surfactant directly down the endotracheal tube.
This will compensate for the meconium-inactivated surfactant.

Start ampicillin and gentamicin.
This will cover the pt until the labs confirm or rule out sepsis.
Inhaled nitric oxide improves oxygenation in pts with meconium aspiration syndrome and pulmonary hypertension.

S **Is there a sibling or parent with congenital heart disease?**
There can be increased risk of recurrence in close relatives.

Does the mother have diabetes or gestational diabetes?
Hyperglycemia can cause congenital heart lesions. Serum glucose should have been kept under control (less than 120) during pregnancy.

Did the mother have any chronic medical problems or use any drugs during pregnancy?
Recreational drugs such as cocaine, amphetamines, or alcohol can be responsible for congenital heart lesions.
The following illnesses and/or their treatments are known to cause congenital heart lesions:

- Lupus	- Hypertension	- Epilepsy	- Atrial fibrillation
- Diabetes	- Acne	- Chronic deep venous thrombosis	

Specific drugs that can cause problems include:

- Lithium	- Isotretinoin	- Warfarin	- Thalidomide

These considerations are especially important during the critical period of heart development (3rd to 7th week of the pregnancy). Many people do not realize they are pregnant this early in the pregnancy.

How old is the mother?
With advanced maternal age, the likelihood of a genetic problem, such as a trisomy, increases.

O **Perform a PE.**
General: Sweating with feeds, generalized cyanosis (not just hands and feet)
Vitals: Tachypnea, tachycardia
Lungs: Shallow respirations, grunting, intercostal retractions, subcostal retractions, nasal flaring, coarse breath sounds
Heart: Unequal peripheral pulses, murmur; extra heart sounds; delayed capillary refill
Look for signs of systemic congenital conditions (Heart Failure p. 20) or inborn errors of metabolism.

Consider more specialized studies.
Chest x-ray
CBC
Perform the hyperoxia test:
ECG
Echocardiogram
- Place on 100% oxygen.
- Check ABG for suggestion of possible right-to-left shunt = $pO_2 < 250$ mm Hg at both pre- and postductal sites.

A **Cyanosis secondary to cardiac causes**
If the infant fails the hyperoxia test, the lesion is very likely dependent on the ductus arteriosus for systemic or pulmonary flow.

Ductal-dependent lesions:
- Transposition of the great vessels — Tricuspid atresia
- Hypoplastic right heart — Ebstein's anomaly
- Pulmonary atresia — Pulmonary stenosis
- Tetralogy of Fallot

- In Tetralogy of Fallot, a ventricular septal defect and a pulmonary valve stenosis caused by an overriding aorta → a hypertrophic right ventricle (four lesions = *tetra*logy).
- In Ebstein's anomaly, displacement of the tricuspid valve down into the R ventricle → large R atrium with a large atrial septal defect (right-to-left shunt) → small R ventricle with poor pulmonary blood flow.

Non-ductal-dependent lesions:
- Total anomalous pulmonary venous connection — Hypoplastic left heart
- Single ventricle — Truncus arteriosus — Common AV canal

Over time, non-ductal-dependent lesions may become ductal dependent.

Noncardiac causes of cyanosis
Neuro: Central hypoventilation, neuromuscular disease, sedation, sepsis
Intraparenchymal lung disease: Pneumonia, aspiration (meconium), respiratory distress syndrome
Airway obstructions: Tracheal stenosis, vascular rings or slings, choanal atresia
Extrinsic lung compression: Pneumothorax, diaphragmatic hernia, pleural effusions
Vascular: Pulmonary AV malformations
Heme/ID: Polycythemia
- Although polycythemia may seem counterintuitive, it is important to understand that 3 to 5 g of deoxygenated hemoglobin result in cyanosis. Thus, if your saturation is 90%, there will be more deoxygenated hemoglobin if the total hemoglobin is 22, than if it is 15. On an ABG, the pO_2 will be normal.

P **Stabilize the pt. Give fluid replacement and pressors. Consider intubation.**

Consider a cardiothoracic surgery consult for congenital heart lesions. If the lesion is ductal dependent, maintain patency of ductus arteriosus with prostaglandin E$_1$ (PGE$_1$).
PGE$_1$ induces vascular muscle relaxation and thus allows the ductus to remain patent.

If PGE$_1$ is not effective, obtain an emergent echocardiogram and plan for possible interventional catheterization for atrial septostomy or valvuloplasty or surgical repair.

For noncardiac cyanotic lesions, consider intubation.
Treat intraparenchymal lung diseases, surgically correct airway obstructions, and relieve external lung compressions (often a chest tube will need to be inserted).
Polycythemic pts may need phlebotomy or exchange transfusions.

S **Is there a sibling or parent with congenital heart disease?**
There is increased risk of occurrence in siblings and children.

Does the mother have a chronic illness, is she of advanced age, or did she use any drugs during pregnancy?
Systemic illnesses and many drugs may have effects on the heart (see Cyanosis p. 18).

O **Do a careful PE looking for signs of heart disease.**
Palpate the precordium and peripheral pulses and auscultate for murmurs or abnormal sounds.
Look for signs of heart failure such as:

- Tachypnea	- Feeding intolerance	- Poor weight gain
- Irritability	- Retractions	- Nasal flaring
- Hepatomegaly	- Edema	

Look for signs of systemic congenital conditions, such as (parentheses indicate the most common associated heart lesion):
Trisomy 13 (ventricular septal defect [VSD]): Cleft lip and palate, low-set ears, polydactyly, aplasia cutis, microcephaly, microphthalmia, holoprosencephaly
Trisomy 18 (VSD): Rocker-bottom feet, clenched fists, overlapping digits, low-set ears, short palpebral fissures, short sternum, prominent occiput
Trisomy 21 (endocardial cushion defects): Upslanting palpebral fissures, midface hypoplasia, large tongue, Simian crease, hypotonia, short fifth finger
Turner syndrome (coarctation of the aorta): Lymphedema of the hands and feet, downslanting palpebral fissures, female, shield chest, low-set ears, short stature, triangular facies, webbed neck, low hairline
Noonan syndrome (pulmonary valve stenosis): Same features as Turner syndrome except can be male. Unlike Turner syndrome, these pts are not genetically monosomy X.
DiGeorge syndrome (interrupted aortic arch): Parathyroid hypoplasia, thyroid hypoplasia, micrognathia, cleft palate, T cell immunodeficiency, thymic hypoplasia
Williams syndrome (supravalvular aortic stenosis): Elfin facies, long philtrum, flat nasal bridge, prominent lips, stellate iris
VACTERL association (VSD): Vertebral anomalies, anal atresia, cardiac defects, tracheoesophageal fistula, renal anomalies, and limb abnormalities

Consider more specialized studies:
CBC with differential, CRP, and blood culture to rule out sepsis
Four extremities BPs to rule out coarctation
Chest x-ray to rule out an enlarged or abnormally shaped heart
ECG looking for arrhythmia, heart block, or chamber hypertrophy
Perform the hyperoxia test (see Cyanosis p. 18)
Echocardiogram

A **Congestive Heart Failure**

The normal course of blood through the heart is Superior and Inferior Vena Cavae →
Right Atrium (*ASD*) → Tricuspid Valve → Right Ventricle (VSD) → Pulmonic Valve
→ Pulmonary Artery (*PDA*) → Lungs → Pulmonary Veins → Left Atrium (*ASD*) →
Mitral Valve → Left Ventricle (VSD) → Aortic Valve → Aorta → Arteries that supply
the upper extremities (*PDA* and Coarctation) → Arteries that supply the lower
extremities → Systemic Vasculature → IVC and SVC.

Consider congenital heart diseases

Outflow obstruction (afterload): Aortic stenosis, aortic coarctation
Left-to-right shunts (preload): Patent ductus arteriosus, aorticopulmonary window,
truncus arteriosus, single ventricle, AV canal, VSD
Although ASD causes a left-to-right shunt, it would be extremely unusual for this
low-pressure system to cause heart failure in infancy.

Consider other causes

Sepsis
Preload: Severe anemia, fluid overload, intracranial AV malformation
Afterload: Hypertension
Contractility: Cardiomyopathy, viral myocarditis, heart block, tachyarrhythmia

P **Consider diuretics for preload lesions.**

Diuretics actually reduce afterload and will make the preload lesions more manageable.

Consider ACE inhibitors for afterload lesions.

Although diuretics are afterload reducers, they will not be effective in the case of
mechanical afterload obstructions. In these cases, vascular resistance must be
decreased.

**Consider dobutamine (acutely) and digoxin (chronically) for
contractility impairment.**

Both of these medications have positive inotropic effects on the heart.

Dopamine may also be used for blood pressure support.

**For critical aortic stenosis, aortic coarctation, aorticopulmonary
window, and truncus arteriosus, consult cardiothoracic surgery as soon
as possible. Critical AS may also be ductal dependent. Consider
prostaglandin E$_1$ to maintain the ductus.**

These lesions can be rapidly fatal and require immediate surgery depending on their
severity.

For patent ductus arteriosus, start indomethacin therapy.

This can be given up to three times before surgical ligation will be required. Term
infants are more likely to require surgery than are preterm infants.

**If the pt has AV canal or ventricular septal defect, treat heart failure
symptoms with diuretics and digoxin and repair electively in the first
year of life. Some VSDs may close spontaneously before surgery is
required.**

S   **Is the baby premature, and what is his or her corrected age?**
Most babies that develop necrotizing enterocolitis (NEC) are born between 30 and
32 weeks' gestational age (WGA). NEC is most likely to occur when the corrected age
is about 34 WGA. That is when a 30 WGA baby is 4 weeks old or a 32 WGA baby is
2 weeks old.
Note that NEC may still occur in term infants.

Did the mother use cocaine during her pregnancy?
Aside from prematurity, cocaine is the only proven risk factor for NEC. It raises the
baby's risk of NEC 2% to 3% presumably by causing vascular damage to the intestines.
Note that other maternal factors, as well as time of year, sex, race, and geography seem
to have no relationship to the risk for NEC.

Do other babies in the NICU have NEC?
NEC seems to occur in clusters. A particular NICU will go months without a case and
then several will occur together.

Has the baby been fed?
About 90% of NEC babies have been started on feeds before developing NEC.
Breast milk is associated with a lower incidence of NEC than formula.

How has the baby been feeding?
Poor feeding, vomiting, and high gastric residual volumes are often found leading up
to NEC.

O   **Examine the baby for signs of NEC.**
Early signs:

- Poor feeding	- Abdominal distention
- Hematochezia	- Decreased bowel sounds

Late signs:

- Irritability	- Abdominal tenderness
- Abdominal erythema	- Respiratory distress
- Ascites	- Apnea
- Bradycardia	- Lethargy

End-stage signs are all signs of shock:

- Hypotension	- Poor perfusion
- Oliguria	- Disseminated intravascular coagulation

Order a kidneys-ureter-bladder (KUB) and cross table lateral x-rays of the abdomen.
Early on, the x-rays will be normal.
Later, you may see the development of an ileus and/or bowel wall edema.
Next, the hallmark of NEC, pneumatosis intestinalis, may become apparent. This
appears as gas inside the bowel wall and looks like thumbprints.
Finally, pneumoperitoneum, a finding indicative of bowel perforation, develops.

Check for grossly bloody stools.
NEC is much more likely to present with grossly bloody stools than occult blood (+)
stools.
If you are notified by nursing of occult blood positivity in the stools, examine the anus
for signs of a fissure, a common neonatal problem. Although a fissure does not rule
out NEC, it will certainly make the occult blood in the stool less concerning.

Review labs for signs of NEC.
Low platelets, low bicarbonate, and low sodium often occurring together.

A **Necrotizing Enterocolitis**
Although no one is entirely sure of the pathophysiology of this disease, it essentially stems from bowel wall ischemia. This is where the three risk factors come into play: (1) prematurity causes immaturity of the intestinal vasculature; (2) cocaine causes intestinal vascular injury; and (3) feeding in this setting may be the final insult for NEC. However, none of these risk factors are required for NEC to occur.

Differential diagnosis:
Neuro: Immature neurologic development leading to poor feeding
Resp: Pneumonia
CV: Heart failure
FEN/GI: Malrotation, intussusception, gastric perforation, diaphragmatic hernia, ileus, anal fissure
Heme/ID: Sepsis, diarrhea

P **Assess the severity of disease, stabilize the pt, draw blood cultures, start antibiotics, and consult a surgeon.**
Bell staging:
  • Stage I: Suspected NEC. Monitor with serial exams and KUBs. Make NPO and start IV antibiotics (ampicillin, gentamicin, and metronidazole) for a minimum of 3 days.
  • Stage II: Definite NEC. Make the pt NPO and continue antibiotics for 10 days.
      - a. Mildly ill   - b. Moderately ill
  • Stage III: Advanced NEC. Critically ill. Maintain NPO and continue antibiotics for 14 days.
      - a. Impending perforation   - b. Proven perforation

Discontinue enteric feedings and place an NG tube with suction to decompress the bowel.
An injured bowel is likely to do very poorly if feeding is continued.

Monitor closely for intestinal perforation or necrosis. Call the surgeon ASAP if it occurs.
Clues may be subtle: Worsening clinical status despite maximal medical therapy, persistent fixed loop on serial KUBs, pneumoperitoneum or air in the biliary tree
In surgery, necrotic bowel is removed and an ostomy is created. Outcome depends on the amount of bowel preserved. Therefore, the earlier the disease is detected, the better.

Assess respiratory status of the pt. Give oxygen and intubate as needed.
A critically ill neonate will have trouble maintaining his or her ventilation.

Assess for hypovolemic or septic shock. Treat with IV fluids and pressor agents as needed.
Signs of shock such as hypotension, tachycardia, oliguria, and poor perfusion will likely occur with intestinal perforation.

Monitor electrolytes and blood sugar, correcting abnormalities as necessary.
Critically ill infants are also likely to have problems with serum chemistries.

Once treated, the pt usually improves within 3 days. If not, consider retained necrotic bowel.

S   **Is the baby yellow?**

Often, the nurse or family member will point out the yellow hue well before you notice it.

How old is the baby?

Usually, the bilirubin level peaks between 60 and 72 hrs of age. Act quickly if it is already high before that, especially in the first 24 hrs. If older than 2 to 3 wks, consider cholestasis.

What is the mother's blood type?

If there is an ABO or Rh incompatibility, immune-mediated hemolysis may occur, leading to an early (within the first 24 hrs) elevated bilirubin and increased risk for kernicterus.

Is the baby breastfed or bottle-fed?

Breastfed babies have two possible reasons to have higher levels of bilirubin:

- *Breast milk jaundice* occurs from an unidentified component of breast milk that leads to slower clearance of bilirubin.
- *Breast-feeding jaundice* occurs in the first few days of life. Because the babies are receiving a relatively small amount of fluids (colostrum versus mature maternal milk), enterohepatic clearance is slowed. This is the more common of the two causes.

Is the baby of Hispanic or Asian descent?

Babies of Asian descent (Native Americans of North, South, and Central America included) have an increased incidence of hyperbilirubinemia.

O   **Examine the baby.**

Look at the baby's skin. The level of jaundice can correlate with the level and intensity of the yellow hue. A light yellow hue of the face is usually a much lower total bilirubin than if the baby is bright yellow/orange to the toes. When visually inspecting for jaundice, try blanching the skin, especially over the nose, with a finger to help reveal the color of the subcutaneous tissues.

Also look carefully for signs of infection, which often causes higher cell turnover and can be the reason for the high bilirubin in the baby.

Check the bilirubin level.

Bilirubin can be either direct (conjugated) or indirect (nonconjugated). Direct is soluble and can therefore be measured. Indirect is not, and therefore cannot. You may obtain a total bilirubin and a direct bilirubin and deduce the indirect by subtraction.

Because conjugation occurs in the liver, indirect hyperbilirubinemia (more common) indicates a prehepatic problem, whereas direct hyperbilirubinemia indicates a posthepatic problem.

A   **Physiologic Jaundice**

Normally, bilirubin levels peak at 60 to 72 hrs of age, so if the baby is discharged before that time, it is important to have rapid follow-up with a pediatrician.

It is helpful to think of jaundice as either an increased production of (secondary to hemolysis) or decreased clearance of bilirubin.

Causes of increased production: Immune-mediated hemolysis, glucose 6 phosphate dehydogenase (G6PD) deficiency, hereditary spherocytosis, abnormal hemoglobin, disseminated intravascular coagulation (DIC)

Causes of decreased clearance: Choledochal cyst, biliary atresia, sepsis, hypothyroidism

Red flags for abnormal jaundice are:

Jaundice before 24 hrs of age

Serum bilirubin increasing by >5 mg/dL/day

Kernicterus

A devastating neurologic disease, occurs when the level of bilirubin is high enough
($>$20-30-mg/dL) such that it crosses the blood–brain barrier. On autopsy, the basal
ganglia are stained yellow.

P   **If jaundiced before 24 hrs, check a Tbili, Coombs, and blood types of
baby and mother.**

Immune-mediated hemolysis is usually maternal in origin. Compare the neonate's
blood type with that of the mother. If the mother is Rh (–) and the baby is Rh (+) or if
they are different ABO types, then it is considered a setup for hemolysis. A positive
Coombs indicates antibodies (maternal IgG) attached to the infant's red blood cells,
causing hemolysis.

**Send a second Tbili to determine the rate of rise of bilirubin. If the
rate of rise or level of Tbili is high ($>$5 mg/dL/day), implement an
exchange transfusion or bili lights depending on severity.**

Kernicterus must be prevented at all costs.

**Consider sepsis and draw a CBC, CRP, and blood culture. Start
antibiotic therapy with ampicillin and gentamicin, and continue them
until sepsis has been ruled out.**

A PT, PTT, LDH, and D-Dimer may also be sent to rule out DIC.

**If jaundiced after 24 hrs and Tbili $>$15 mg/dL, start bili lights
(phototherapy).**

It has long been known that insoluble bilirubin can be chemically inactivated (and
made soluble) by ultraviolet light. There is enough UV light in the visible light
spectrum to decrease the pt's serum bilirubin concentration if placed under bright
light.

**If Tbili $>$20 mg/dL or rising faster than 0.5 mg/dL/hr, perform an
exchange transfusion.**

The rate of rise is best tracked by plotting out the baby's Tbilis on a graph with the
y-axis as Tbili and the x-axis as time.

An exchange transfusion attempts to remove antibody-coated RBCs and replace them
with immunologically inactive ones to decrease the rate of immune-mediated
hemolysis. It is more effective than phototherapy but also carries significantly
increased risk to the pt.

**If the pt is not improving, consider checking a thyroid-stimulating
hormone, hemoglobin electrophoresis, and testing for G6PD
deficiency and hereditary spherocytosis.**

These will help rule out the more rare causes of jaundice.

**If Dbili $>$20% of Tbili, image the right upper quadrant with ultrasound
or CT.**

It is rare for biliary obstruction to present in the NICU, but if Dbili is high, it must be
ruled out.

**If the pt is jaundiced after 2 wks of age, consider causes of cholestatic
jaundice, especially if not breastfeeding. Ask about dark urine or
light-colored stools. Check for hepatomegaly and a direct bilirubin. If
clinical suspicion is high, image the right upper quadrant.**

If the pt does develop biliary atresia, a good outcome would be more likely if a
hepatointestinal anastamosis (Kasai procedure) is performed as soon as possible.
Therefore, time should not be wasted in attempting to make a diagnosis.

S **What maternal risk factors for sepsis does this baby have?**

Learn the risk factors of the pt as soon as possible because the septic workup should begin at the resuscitation if the pt has risk factors or symptoms.

Maternal risk factors include:

- Premature labor (<37 wks): Infection is thought to be a cause of premature delivery.
- Prolonged rupture of membranes (>18 hrs)
- Maternal vaginal or urethral colonization with group B streptococcus (GBS)
- Peripartum infection, either sepsis or chorioamnionitis: Often the only intrapartum indication of this is peripartum fever (temp > 37.5°C).
- Previous baby with invasive GBS disease

What neonatal risk factors for sepsis are present?

Low birth weight

A neonate weighing less than 2500 g is at a greater risk for sepsis and meningitis.

Was this mother screened for GBS and, if so, was she treated?

Intrapartum ampicillin effectively prevents GBS infections, so rectal and vaginal swabs are collected at 35 to 37 wks' gestation for GBS. If either the cultures or the risk factors listed above are positive, the mother should receive intrapartum penicillin G or ampicillin.

Penicillin-allergic mothers may have been treated with clindamycin or erythromycin.

O **Does the pt have any clinical signs of sepsis?**

No signs: Clinical signs may be subtle; occasionally there will be no clinical signs at all.

Vital signs: Fevers (normal: 36°C to 37°C), hypothermia, hypotension

- Preterm neonates are more likely to be hypothermic, whereas term neonates are more likely to have a fever.

Neurologic signs: Lethargy, seizures, irritability

Respiratory signs: Up to 90% of all septic infants will have respiratory distress; shallow respirations, grunting, intercostal retractions, subcostal retractions, nasal flaring, apneas

Cardiovascular signs: Sweating with feeds, tachycardia, poor perfusion

Gastrointestinal signs: Intrauterine passage of meconium, vomiting, diarrhea, abdominal distention, poor feeding

Renal signs: Decreased urine output

Hematologic signs: Pallor or jaundice

Skin signs: Petechiae and purpura

What lab studies should be done?

Order a CBC with differential and a blood culture. Also consider a CRP.

A CBC is considered positive if the WBC count is <5, the total neutrophil count is less than 1000, or if the band neutrophil to total neutrophil ratio is greater than 0.2.

A blood culture is considered positive if it grows a pathologic organism. In neonates, even coagulase-negative staphylococcus can be a pathogen (it may also be a contaminant).

An elevated CRP is supportive of the CBC and blood culture.

Should a lumbar puncture be done?

This policy may differ by facility, but in general it has been found that a lumbar puncture should be done only if the pt is going to receive antibiotic treatment (and is stable enough to tolerate the procedure). If you are performing an LP, send the cerebrospinal fluid (CSF) for culture, gram stain, cell count, glucose, protein, and any special studies to diagnose diseases you may be suspicious for, such as herpes or TB. See Fever with Irritability (p. 92) for normal and abnormal CSF values.

A Rule out sepsis.

Neonates have not yet developed their immune systems, and their blood–brain barriers are not as strong as those of adults. Therefore, they are unable to properly contain infections, and significant morbidity and mortality can result. Since rule out sepsis protocols have been implemented, morbidity and mortality have been markedly decreased. Therefore, when in doubt, treat.

The most likely pathogens are the following:

Group B streptococcus is the most common etiology, followed by *E. coli*. Other pathogens include nontypeable *H. influenzae*, Enterococcus, *Listeria monocytogenes*, *Citrobacter diversus*, and nosocomial infections such as *Staphylococcus aureus* and coagulase-negative staphylococcus (especially if the pt has any indwelling catheters).

Documented sepsis actually occurs between 1 and 8 cases per 1000 live births. One-third of all cases progress to meningitis.

P Draw a CBC with differential, CRP, and blood culture on all pts with suspected sepsis. This is the rule out sepsis workup.

Mild maternal risk factors but no symptoms or signs

Consider starting ampicillin and gentamicin and treating for at least 3 days.

These agents will cover just about all of the pathogens noted above.

If the mother has (+) GBS cultures, or unknown GBS status, and multiple risk factors, she should have received intrapartum antibiotics at least 4 hrs before delivery. If she did not, after the labs are drawn, and the LP is performed, begin antibiotics.

Also treat if the pt has mild respiratory distress or other symptoms.

Stop antibiotics after 3 days if the PE and labs are negative.
Consider continuing treatment for 7 to 14 days for the following:

Symptomatic with fevers, respiratory distress, etc.

Any part of the CBC, blood cultures, CRP, suggests infection.

If meningitis is present on the LP results, increase doses and continue for 14 to 21 days. GBS proven sepsis by positive culture requires treatment with penicillin.

S **What type of diabetes does the mother have and how is it controlled?**
Gestational (insulin or diet-controlled): Onset during pregnancy
Class A (diet-controlled): Diagnosed before pregnancy
Class B (insulin-dependent diabetes): Onset >20 yrs old and duration <10 yrs
Class C_1: Onset 10 to 19 yrs old
        C_2: Duration 10 to 19 yrs
Class D_1: Onset before 10 yrs old
        D_2: Duration $\geq$20 yrs

Does she have any other comorbid conditions?
Class F: Nephropathy with proteinuria over 500 mg per day
Class R: Proliferative retinopathy or vitreous hemorrhage
Class G: Many spontaneous abortions/fetal demises
Class H: Evidence of coronary artery disease
Class T: Status post-renal transplant

What was the average blood sugar during pregnancy?
To reduce or avoid complications, blood sugar should be kept below 120 during
  pregnancy.

What is the gestational age of the baby?
The younger the baby, the higher the risk of such diagnoses as respiratory distress
  syndrome (RDS) and hyperbilirubinemia. Infants of diabetic mothers (IDMs) are
  associated with an increased risk of RDS, and generally, because they make glycemic
  control more difficult, corticosteroids (which would normally hasten fetal lung
  maturation) are not given.

Was an U/S done?
Given the increased risk of fetal macrosomia or congenital malformations such as
  sacral agenesis and anencephaly, it is good to have an U/S at about 18 wks and then
  again at 28 wks.

O **Look carefully for signs of distress:**
Remember the increased risk of RDS and hypoglycemia. Signs of distress include:
        - Shallow respirations   - Grunting   - Intercostal retractions
        - Subcostal retractions   - Nasal flaring   - Apneas

Do a PE and observe carefully for possible fetal anomalies
IDMs have increased anomalies of the central nervous system (CNS), heart, skeleton,
  GI tract, and urinary system. Macrosomia is the most common physical anomaly.

Check glucose, hematocrit, calcium, magnesium, and bilirubin, and consider a sepsis workup with CBC, CRP, and blood culture.
Because of pancreatic islet hypertrophy, IDMs can have hypoglycemia. Glucose should
  be checked on arrival to the NICU and before each successive feed (q3h) × 2.
Polycythemia is common.
Hypocalcemia and hypomagnesemia can be associated with hyperinsulinism.
IDMs are at increased risk for jaundice secondary to polycythemia and poor liver
  function.
Sepsis is more common in these babies secondary to poor initial immune system
  function.

Check a chest x-ray and consider a kidneys-ureter-bladder/ echocardiogram for abnormalities.
As mentioned above, many skeletal, heart, GU, and GI tract abnormalities can occur in these infants.

Infants of Diabetic Mothers
Blood sugars consistently greater than 120 in utero can cause many problems for the neonate. Typically, babies are born large for their gestational age but are neurologically immature and behave as preemies. Many systems may not form correctly. The most common problems are:

- Macrosomia   - Meningocele   - Cardiac abnormalities
- Sacral agenesis   - Vertebral anomalies   - Small left colon
- Colonic atresia   - Islet cell hypertrophy - Sepsis

Macrosomia leads to a higher incidence of birth trauma, such as fractured clavicle, Erb's palsy, and shoulder dystocia. See Birth Trauma (p. 4).

Look specifically for the common lab derangements:
- Hypoglycemia   - Hypocalcemia
- Polycythemia   - Jaundice

P If the baby is asymptomatic, carefully follow the blood sugars and how well the baby feeds. Then, if everything goes well, the baby can go to the normal newborn nursery.
Treatment greatly depends on what is wrong with the baby. This action is only to prevent the most common problem in these pts, which is hypoglycemia secondary to islet cell hypertrophy. If they do well with this, nothing else needs to be done.

Check to make sure that the infant is feeding well
IDMs have many possible causes of poor feeding:
- CNS immaturity   - Cardiac lesion   - Respiratory difficulty
- Phrenic nerve injury - Diaphragmatic hernia   - Colonic atresia

If hypoglycemic, start IV glucose with D10 or D25W or D10 calcium gluconate.
About 40% of IDMs develop hypocalcemia between 24 and 72 hrs, so calcium gluconate may be required.

Check calcium and magnesium and replace as necessary.
A low calcium will not resolve until hypomagnesemia is corrected.

Do not treat polycythemia unless the hematocrit is >70% (asymptomatic) or >65% (symptomatic).
The excess RBCs will self-correct shortly.

Treat jaundice as you would in any other infant (see Jaundice p. 24).
Hyperbilirubinemia is also common in the younger gestational age IDMs.

Congenital anomalies such as meningomyelocele, sacral agenesis, colonic atresia, or cardiac abnormalities may need surgical consult/correction.

Is there advance knowledge that the mother of the pt is a substance abuser and, if so, of what substances?

The condition is much easier to diagnose if it is already expected. Different substances tend to have different withdrawal profiles and different long-term effects. In order to properly treat these infants, it is beneficial to have advance knowledge of their conditions.

If there is denial of drug use, is there any other reason to suspect it?

Maternal conditions that are associated with substance abuse include:

- Early labor	- Rapid delivery	- Placental rupture/abruption
- Prostitution	- No prenatal care	- Tuberculosis
- Hepatitis B	- Hepatitis C	- HIV

Is the mother taking any legal medications that can have behavioral effects on the neonate?

Medications that can cause abnormal behaviors in the baby include:

- Phenothiazines	- Tricyclic antidepressants	- Antihistamines
- Benzodiazepines	- Barbiturates	

Was there neonatal respiratory depression in the delivery room? Was naloxone required?

A neonate with respiratory depression in the delivery room implies recent use of narcotics. These can be given by the obstetricians during labor, but check the delivery records to be sure.

Response to Narcan (naloxone) definitely suggests opiate intoxication.

Does the neonate have any gross physical signs of being an infant of a substance-abusing mother (ISAM)?

Being small for gestational age or microcephalic implies the hypoxia/placental insufficiency associated with cocaine and nicotine.

Far more rarely, neonatal stroke or arterial infarction (leading to congenital defects such as intestinal atresia) also imply use of the same two vasoconstricting substances.

Features consistent with fetal alcohol syndrome include:

- Hydronephrosis	- Microcephaly	- Small for gestational
- Low nasal bridge	- Flattened philtrum	age
- Hypoplastic midface	- Epicanthal folds	- Thin upper lip
- Heart lesions		- Shortened palpebral fissure

What are the pt's vital signs?

Narcotic withdrawal: Fever, tachypnea, tachycardia
Benzodiazepine and alcohol withdrawal: Tachypnea
Tricyclic antidepressant withdrawal: Tachypnea and tachycardia
A febrile pt should also begin antibiotics and receive a septic workup. See Rule Out Sepsis/Meningitis (p. 26).

What behavioral and neurologic signs of withdrawal are present?

Behavioral: Ineffective suck, increased suck, sneezing/yawning, altered sleep-wake cycle, lethargy, high-pitched cry, irritability, increased appetite
Neurologic: Vomiting, diarrhea, seizures, sweating, cyanosis, tremors, hypertonicity, hypotonicity, hyperreflexia, jitteriness
Other: Nasal congestion, abdominal distention, weight loss

Perform a urine toxicology screen.
This may be done on the neonate and the mother. It will be the simplest way to tell if your pt was exposed to a controlled substance.
It is important to point out that in a symptomatic infant, there is no need for parental consent to perform the screen. This can be justified as diagnosis and treatment of a suspected medical condition. However, in an asymptomatic infant in whom there is suspicion because of corresponding maternal factors noted above, it may be considered unethical to screen without parental consent. In some states it is illegal to do so.
In either case, it is always a good idea to keep the parent informed, because the results of the screen may lead to the pt being taken from the mother (see below).

If the pt is known to be an ISAM, and maternal HIV and HBV status are not known, they should be followed up! Your pt may be at risk for a preventable infectious disease.

A

Infant of a Substance-Abusing Mother
It is always important to know if your pt is an ISAM because most substances of abuse can cross the placenta and have a profound effect on the fetus. Some of these may require treatment and some may not. Most will have important social implications.

Differential diagnosis
Neonates may have a CNS defect caused by their mothers' substance abuse that leads to seizures. They may have an infection that leads to jitteriness and seizures. As always in the NICU, rule out sepsis.

Long-Term Complications
Most of the potentially abused substances can have long-term complications that include increased incidence of attention deficit hyperactivity disorder, learning disabilities, flat, apathetic moods, and mental retardation. It is also important to point out that narcotics, cocaine, and tobacco also increase the risk of sudden infant death syndrome.

P

Treat the infant's withdrawal symptoms. Start with nonpharmacologic treatment.
It includes tight swaddling, holding, rocking, and placing the baby in a slightly darkened, quiet area. You can also try using a hypercaloric (24 kcal/ounce) formula. Nonpharmacologic treatment will be effective approximately 40% of the time.

For opioid withdrawal, start pharmacologic treatment with mild opioid solutions, including neonatal morphine, tincture of opium, methadone, and paregoric. Use tapering doses.
Phenobarbital or lorazepam may also be effective.

For cocaine withdrawal, consider starting phenobarbital or lorazepam for sedation.
Other controlled substances generally have no prescribed treatment for withdrawal.

Notify Social Services.
Many of these pts will require placement. Remember, these children tend to be difficult, as was stated above. They will try a caregiver's patience and are at an increased risk for abuse.

III

Pediatric Clinic

S **Ask developmental questions appropriate for age for each visit.**

1 week: Visually fixes

1 month: Raises head slightly from prone, tight grasp, alerts to sound, regards face

2 months: Raises chest off table, smiles, recognizes parents, relaxes grasp

4 months: Rolls front to back, coos/laughs, explores visually, hands midline

6 months: Rolls back to front/sits, raking grasp, recognizes stranger, babbles

9 months: Says "mama/dada"/gestures, pincer grasp, holds bottle/throws, cruises

12 months: Says "mama/dada" (specific), walks, comes when called, three-word vocabulary

What is the baby eating? How often is the mother feeding?

Exclusively breastfeeding q 2–3 hrs is best for the baby until about 6 months, then start baby food and water. Breastfeeding may be continued as long as the mother feels comfortable.

For bottle/formula feeding, from 1 wk to 6 months should take up to 3 ounces every 3 hrs. At 6 to 12 months, give no more than 4 ounces every 3 hrs to allow for adequate intake of solid foods.

How many diapers per day? How many with stool?

Stool: Initially occurs after every feed (q 2–3 hrs for breastfeeding and q 3–4 hrs for bottle-feeding). As the infant approaches 1 year, stooling will become less frequent (about 1/day).

Urine: About 8 wet diapers per day. If significantly less, consider dehydration or urinary tract infection.

How is the baby sleeping?

Newborns sleep about 15 hrs per day, sleeping only a few hours at a time.

By about 4 months, they should be able to sleep through the night (about 5 hrs at a time).

By 12 months, they should sleep about 14 hrs a day (10 hrs/night and two naps during the day).

O **Perform a PE, making sure to include the following:**

Growth parameters: Weight, height, and head circumference should be plotted on a growth curve so as to not miss malnutrition, failure to thrive, or poor brain growth.

Fontanelles: Posterior closes at about 2 months, anterior closes at about 18 months.

Eyes: Looking for leukocoria (white instead of red reflex). Differential diagnosis: retinoblastoma or cataracts.

Infant Neuro Exam:

- Tone: Hypertonic (CP), normal, or hypotonic (CP, botulism, metabolic disorder)
- Primitive reflexes: Palmar grasp, Moro, Gallant, and Perez = birth to 3–6 months
- Plantar grasp and ATNR (fencer response) = birth to 4–9 months
- Postural reactions: Head righting and Landau by 3 months, derotational righting by 5 months, parachute by 6 months, Ant/Lat/Post Propping by 5, 6, and 7 months, respectively.

Hip clunks: **O**rtolani (**O**ut) and **B**arlow (**B**ack) (see Newborn Exam p. 2).

Umbilical cord: Should have fallen off by 1 month. If not, consider leukocyte/neutrophil defect.

Testes down bilaterally: Abdominal testes have increased risk of testicular cancer.

A **Well Infant, Age:** _____
Assess development.

Some diagnoses to consider while assessing developmental delay are cerebral palsy, hearing deficit (poor language development), and autism (poor social and language development).

Assess appropriateness of growth.

Newborns weigh approximately 3 kg; they lose and then regain birth weight by 7 to 10 days of age. Most weigh approximately 10 kg by 1 year. Plot the height, weight, and head circumference. If any of them is below the 5th percentile or the current plot is not following the expected growth curve, this should be investigated further.

P **Give anticipatory guidance. Recommend contacting the doctor if there is:**

Runny nose/congestion that interferes with breathing

Prolonged fatigue or irritability

Vomiting and decreased oral intake

Audible wheezing

Diarrhea and dehydration

Fever in an infant younger than 1 month of age

Offer appropriate anticipatory guidance related to the safety of the infant's environment:

- No unlocked guns in the home
- All possible poisons out of reach
- Electric outlet protectors
- Infants should not be left in the bath alone (they can drown and die in as little as 1 inch of water).
- Smoke detectors
- Prevent falls
- Reset water heater to 120°F

Give appropriate vaccinations.

Because the regimens change regularly, and many combination vaccines with different administration schedules are available, it is best to find the most recent version of the vaccination schedule at www.cispimmunize.org.

Recommend exclusive breastfeeding (bottle-feeding as a second choice) until about 6 months.

Endorse breastfeeding because there is no better food for the baby.

Before 6 months, reserve solid food for smaller babies. Feeding earlier increases risk of food allergies.

At 6 months, recommend introducing baby food and the cup.

Start rice cereal first for about a week, then begin introducing new strained or pureed foods a week at a time, vegetables, then fruits, then meats.

With the cup, the bottle should be phased out and water and juice introduced.

At 8 to 10 months, recommend starting things in small pieces such as:

Cereal, pasta, banana, crackers, cooked chicken, and vegetables

Discuss foods to avoid before 1 yr of age:

Honey because of the risk of infant botulism

Foods that the baby can choke on, such as hot dogs (these are okay if you cut them length-wise in thin strips), nuts, seeds, popcorn, chips, grapes, raisins, raw vegetables, and peanut butter

Potential allergens, such as egg whites, milk, orange juice, nuts, strawberries, tomatoes, and fish

Check CBC and lead level at the 1-yr visit to rule out anemia or lead ingestion.

S During a well child visit, you should always start off by asking how the child is doing.

In addition to any complaints, be sure to assess eating, sleeping, stooling, and voiding.

Obtain a developmental history.

Use a Denver Developmental Survey form for developmental assessment. Remember that the Denver test only screens for delay. Even if the child "fails" the Denver test, he or she may still be completely normal.

The Denver test varies considerably from American Academy of Pediatrics (AAP) sources, so we recommend studying AAP sources (see Table 2) for your exams.

Failure to reach these milestones appropriately are red flags.

Screen for exposure to lead, smoking, domestic violence, and guns in the home.

Table 2 Developmental Assessment			
	18 months	**24 months**	**36 months**
Gross Motor	Walks fast; runs; walks up stairs; throws a ball	Runs well; walks down stairs; kicks a ball	Walks up stairs on toes; uses tricycle (3 yrs = 3 wheels); hops on 1 foot
Fine Motor	Builds a tower of 4 cubes; scribbles spontaneously; copies a vertical line	Builds a tower of 6 to 7 cubes; copies a horizontal line; uses a spoon with less spilling	Builds a tower of 9 to 10 cubes; draws a head; copies a circle
Social/ Emotional	Takes off clothes; feeds self (spills); hugs a doll	Refers to self by name; says when needs the toilet; plays in parallel	Shows concern for others; plays cooperatively; dresses with help
Language	Follows two-step commands; looks at book; names one object; says 10 to 20 words	Uses 2- to 3-word phrases; 150- to 200-word vocabulary; uses "I" "me" "you"; 25% to 50% intelligible	75% intelligible; 4- to 5-word phrases; tells stories
Intellectual	Understands cause and effect; points to named body parts; understands object permanence	Solve by trial and error; understands time	Asks "why?"; recites rhymes; follows daily routine

O Check the toddler's height, weight, and head circumference.

Height should increase by 12.5 cm over the second year of life and 6.25 cm over the third. The child should gain about 5 to 8 g per day.

Head circumference should continue to be followed until age 36 months.

Plot on growth curve. If not in normal range or growth rate decreasing, investigate.

Perform a PE.

Usually, a child younger than 3 yrs old continues to experience stranger anxiety.

Examine the chest first so that you may be able to auscultate before the child begins to cry. Then examine the abdomen, extremities, and genitalia. The abdomen softens and can be palpated when the child inhales to cry.

The exam of the head, ears, eyes, nose, and throat should be done with the child seated in mother's lap. Mother should hold both of the child's hands in one hand, and use her other hand to hold the head, which prevents sudden movements during the exam.

If the child bites down on the tongue blade, slide it slowly and gently forward. When the gag reflex is triggered, the child will open the mouth and you may examine the throat.

A Well Toddler, Age: _____
Consider the following possible complicating diagnoses, which may present in this period:
Gross/fine motor abnormalities: Cerebral palsy, hypothyroidism, muscular dystrophy
Social/emotional/language failures: Autism, hearing impairment, mental retardation
Intellectual failures: Consider mental retardation
Obesity: Calculate the BMI = (weight in kg) ÷ (height in m)^2, plot it on the BMI curve, and if pt is obese or at risk of obesity, address this issue with the family. Be aggressive because obesity will significantly shorten children's lives.
Failure to thrive: If the child is not gaining weight, this should be investigated as well. Both social and medical causes should be considered.
Evaluate for medical conditions related to the complaint of the parents or child.

P Give anticipatory guidance. Advise the parents on the following safety issues:
Climbing risks, falling risks, ingestion risks (both chemical and foreign body)
Pool should be gated (if there is one).
Lock up cleaning supplies or place them in unreachable areas.
Lock up all guns with ammunition locked away separately.
Adult supervision is needed while the child is near or crossing the street (driveways, ice cream trucks, exiting car).

Advise the parents on toilet training techniques, including:
Positive reward systems, a special potty chair, and to avoid making it a struggle, which usually ends in constipation.

Advise the parents on discipline for temper tantrums, especially the timeout method.
Studies have shown that timeouts are more effective at decreasing tantrums than corporal punishment. Spanking, although tolerated, is no longer advised. (See WCC: Child p. 38).

Advise decreased bottle use and minimized juice intake.
The bottle is bad for the toddler's teeth. Juice has little nutritional value and leads to obesity.

Vaccinate for DTaP at 15 months and Hep A at 2 yrs with a repeat in 6 months. Check lead level (for toxicity), CBC (for anemia), and U/A if none in last 2 yrs.
Anemia is very common and is usually secondary to increased milk intake. Advise no more than 16 oz of milk per day.

For milestone failures, follow-up in 3 months to check for milestone attainment.
Screen the hearing for all language failures. If failure persists, refer to a child developmental specialist or your local Social Services center for support.

S Begin with a typical open-ended question about whether there are any problems, and then move to developmental questions that are appropriate for the child's age.

4 years: Balances on one foot for 3 seconds, alternates feet going down steps, uses all utensils (except knife), can name colors, understands concept of past, speech 100% intelligible, speaks in paragraphs, can draw a plus sign, buttons

5 years: Balances on one foot for 10 seconds, can jump over low obstacles, ties shoes, spreads with knife, competitive play, asks for definitions, can draw a square

6 years: Counts to ten, knows right from left, can draw a triangle

8 years: Sounds out words, can print name, can draw a diamond

10 years: Tells time, does chores, does well in school

What is the child eating?

Explain that it is the parent's job to offer a balanced diet (limit junk food) and the child's job to select from among the options. It is very common for parents to think that their children don't eat enough. As long as the child is growing normally (confirm by plotting the child's growth curve), everything will be fine.

If the child is obese, this question will help you learn what foods may be easy to eliminate.

Ask how things are going at home, school, and in the child's outside activities.

Problems in one or all of these areas will give you reason to investigate things such as domestic violence, discipline, and learning disabilities.

Ask questions related to the safety of the home environment.

Ask specifically about smoke alarms (and whether there are functioning batteries), and if there are guns, violence, drugs, or tobacco in the home.

O Review and plot growth parameters on a growth chart.

It is important to plot not only height and weight but also to calculate body mass index (BMI: weight in kg/[height in cm]^2) because many children are obese, and it is important to recognize its severity when you see it. If the BMI is around 20 or greater, the child is at risk of obesity. If the BMI is more than 25, the child is obese.

Watch how the child and parents interact.

You may see clues to make you consider discipline problems, ADHD, or even child abuse.

Perform a PE. Order appropriate tests as necessary.

If you assess delayed development or school problems, a hearing and vision screen would be an appropriate first step.

If you pick up scoliosis on PE, you should check an x-ray of the spine.

Check a urinalysis at 5 yrs old to rule out occult UTI or insidious onset of proteinuria secondary to such renal conditions as focal segmental glomerulosclerosis, which commonly presents at this age.

A **Well Child, Age:** _____
Assess the development of child.
If you assess delay, check hearing and vision and consider conditions such as autism and ADHD.
Assess the safety of the home environment.
If any of the answers to the questions you asked above indicate an unsafe environment, such as guns, violence, drugs, or lack of smoke detectors in the home, give appropriate anticipatory guidance.
Assess whether pt is obese.
As described above, this is becoming a very common problem. In the 1970s, about 4% of children in this age group were obese; by 2000, it had more than tripled to 15%.

P **Give anticipatory guidance.**
Change from car seat to booster seat for car lap and shoulder belt at 108 cm (about 43 inches = 50% for 5-yr-old).
Remove booster seat at 136 cm (about 54 inches = 50% for 10-yr-old).
Safety helmets for bikes, roller-blades, skates, scooters, etc.
Crossing the street safely is very important because pedestrians versus automobiles is a common reason for admission. All children should be supervised by an adult while crossing the street.
Water safety: There should always be a fence around pools and an adult supervising.

Recommend exercise or some sort of physical activity.
Limit junk food, desserts, sodas, and chips to prevent obesity when the BMI is ≥20.
Limit TV time to prevent inactivity, snacking, obesity, and improve interaction with the family.
Brush twice a day and floss nightly and visit a dentist to prevent tooth decay.

Discuss why hitting children for punishment is wrong.
It sends the wrong message that hitting and being hit is okay. A more effective method is the timeout. When the child misbehaves, say "Timeout, hitting" or whatever short phrase that is applicable and calmly remove the child from the environment, isolating him or her (facing a wall, corner, or any other uninteresting place) until the time has been completed. Because of the limited attention span of children, the timeout should last about 1 minute for each year of life. Timeouts can be used repeatedly without any harm to the child.

Discuss sex education.
It is always better for the parents to address this issue in the prepubertal age before any of the child's friends who think they are experts on the subject get to them first.
Puberty/Menarche: Prepubertal girls should know what menses is before it happens.
Discuss the use of money.
Children in this age group should be given supervised opportunities to use money.
Discuss school readiness.
If a learning, hearing, or vision problem is detected, it should be addressed before it interferes with school.
Discuss drugs, tobacco, and alcohol and the dangers of using them.
As with sex education, it is best to demystify this topic in the doctor's office rather than on the school playground.
Give appropriate vaccinations.
DTaP, IPV, and MMR should be given at 4 yrs old, before starting school.

S **If the parent is present, begin the interview with the parent and adolescent together. After discussing the parent's concerns, ask her or him to wait in the waiting room.**

Talk to adolescents alone so they can talk about things they do not want their parents to hear.

Explain that confidentiality is broken only to prevent serious harm to someone.

Remember to use open-ended questions and the mnemonic HEADDSS:

H (Home): How are things at home?
Ask about: Live with parents, friends, homeless; physical, sexual, verbal abuse; discipline

E (Education): How is school?
Ask about: Grade level, performance, goals; detention, truancy, expulsion; learning difficulties

A (Activities): What do you do when you're not in school?
Ask about: Jobs, what they do for money; sports, hobbies, clubs; gangs, arrests

D (Diet): What do you normally eat?
Ask about: Number of meals per day, junk food; using laxatives, vomiting

D (Drugs): Do you use any drugs?
Ask about: Alcohol (how much, what kind); smoking (packs per day, how many yrs); illicit drugs

S (Sex): Are you having sex?
Ask about: Age at first intercourse; age and sex of partner; use of contraception; type of sex (vaginal, rectal, oral); number of partners; condom, dental dams; STDs, discharge, genital lesions; sex for money, housing, or food; unwanted sex

S (Suicide): Do you feel depressed? Do you ever feel like hurting yourself?
A good mnemonic for depression is SIG E CAPS:

- Sleep (insomnia or oversleeping)
- Interest (less for normal activities)
- Guilt
- Energy (lack of)
- Concentration (lack of)
- Attention (lack of)
- Psychomotor agitation (nervous activity)
- Suicidal thoughts

If they have thought of hurting themselves, ask about SLAP (Suicidal, Lethality, Attempts/Access, Plan):

- Suicidal thoughts currently
- Access to lethal means
- Lethality of plan
- Plan about how to do it
- Previous Attempts

Do they have thoughts of hurting or killing someone else? If so, do they have current plans?

O **Perform a general PE.**
This can be done with the parent present or absent, depending on the adolescent's choice.

If sexually active, perform a genital exam (including pap smear for women) with chaperone.

Check growth and development.
Note rapid increases in weight or decreases in height velocity.

Assess sexual development (breast, pubic hair, genital) by Tanner Sexual Maturity Rating:
- I: No breast development or pubic hair, prepubertal testes

- II: Breast bud diameter < areolar, sparse thin pubic hair
- III: Breast bud diameter > areolar, sparse coarse pubic hair, penis lengthens. Menarche for girls usually occurs after Tanner Stage III.
- IV: Mounding of areola, coarse hair confined to mons, penis grows in width
- V: Adult breast development, pubic hair extending to thigh, adult testes

If breast enlargement (gynecomastia) found in males, reassure that it's normal and will resolve.

Perform a U/A and test all sexually active teens for sexually transmitted infections (STIs).

Test all sexually active teens at risk for STIs and perform a U/A (+ leukocyte esterase enzyme on the dipstick may indicate occult chlamydial infection).

A

Adolescents should also be assessed for:

Pubertal delay or short stature: If there are no signs of sexual development by age 14, investigate chromosomal or endocrine causes.

Home problems: From abuse to homelessness

School problems: From learning difficulties to behavior problems

Eating disorders: Anorexia, bulimia, or obesity

Risk-taking behaviors: Such as substance abuse, reckless driving, unprotected sex, homelessness

Suicidal ideation: Caused by problems at home, abuse, or clinical depression

Scoliosis and any other general medical problems

P

Anticipatory guidance and counseling.

It is extremely helpful for the teen to hear advice from a nonparental authority figure.

Home problems: Investigate abuse and take appropriate measures depending on severity.

Learning problems: Offer a referral to the appropriate school services assessment. Behavior problems: Identify the source of the problem, such as abuse or influence of friends.

If you suspect apathetic effort, try to counsel on the importance of education.

Counsel the teen regarding dangerous activities, such as gangs, that may lead to arrest.

Diet: Counsel regarding problems with obesity, anorexia, or bulimia.

All will significantly shorten the adolescent's life.

Drugs: Assess for alcohol, smoking, and drug use. Offer a referral to programs such as Alcoholics Anonymous or other rehabilitative programs. Counsel on the dangers of the following:

Alcohol: Cirrhosis, varices

Smoking: Cancer, chronic obstructive pulmonary disease

Drugs: Overdose, HIV, hepatitis

Sex: Assess for high-risk behaviors and counsel on the risk of pregnancy, dangers of STIs (HIV, herpes, etc.), and offer testing, treatment, barrier methods (condoms, dental dams), and contraception.

Give the dT (diphtheria, tetanus) shot if longer than 10 yrs since last DTaP (usually >13 yrs).

Return to clinic in 1 yr, or sooner if indicated by above possible social problems.

S   What symptoms does your child have?

Hyperactivity: Leaving his or her seat in class, running or climbing at inappropriate times, fidgeting, squirming, talking excessively

Attention deficit: Frequent careless errors, not listening when spoken to directly, not finishing schoolwork or chores, losing things necessary for tasks (like schoolwork), obvious distraction by extraneous stimuli

Impulsivity: Blurting out answers before questions are asked, not waiting his or her turn, interrupting others

What is the child's sex?

Attention deficit hyperactivity disorder (ADHD) is far more common in male than female children in up to a 9:1 ratio.

How old is the child?

The child should be school age. Toddlers who act in the aforementioned manner are acting age appropriately. Just because the parents are exasperated does not mean the child has ADHD.

Teens with onset of these symptoms may be using mind-altering drugs that might be responsible for their behavior. They may also be developing an oppositional disorder. If symptoms were not present by age 7 years, the child is unlikely to have ADHD.

Does the child have symptoms in more than one setting?

Hyperactivity just at school or just at home does not count as ADHD.
ADHD must be pervasive in more than one setting.

How long have the symptoms been going on?

In order to diagnose ADHD, symptoms have to have been present for at least 6 months.

Obtain a birth history.

Risk factors for ADHD include:
- Maternal substance abuse   - Low APGAR scores   - Prematurity

Does the child take any medicines?

The following medications can cause symptoms that mimic ADHD:
- Beta-agonists   - Theophylline   - Phenobarbital

Is there a family history of ADHD, learning disability, tics, obsessive compulsive disorder, or Tourette's syndrome?

The gene loci for these problems are very close, and 70% to 80% of the problems that cause ADHD are genetic. An example is Fragile X syndrome, a common genetic cause of ADHD.

O   Observe the child in the clinic while you are obtaining the History.

As noted above, symptoms of hyperactivity or impulsiveness should be present in more than one setting. That may include the clinic.

Perform a general PE including a detailed neurologic exam.

The child may be excessively clumsy and do poorly on the neuro exam. This includes poor finger-to-nose, sliding heel on shin, rapid alternating movements, and an inability to walk heel to toe. These are neurologic "soft signs," but in this case they are extremely significant.

Also check the child's kinesthetic sense: ability to recognize a paper clip by touch or telling the difference in size between a penny and a quarter.

On the PE, be sure to check for physical signs of a genetic disorder. Fragile X presents with long facies, prominent ears, and large testicles.

Perform the test of attention preferred by your hospital or facility.
Multiple tests of attention exist, including the TOVA, the IVA, the Stroop Color Word Test, and the Wisconsin Card Sort Test.

Refer for an EEG.
There may be fairly nonspecific abnormalities in ADHD; however, this will be diagnostic if you suspect your pt has absence seizures. These pts exhibit a three-per-second spike and wave pattern on the EEG. This is characteristic of absence or petit mal seizures.

A **Rule Out ADHD.**
Per the DSM-IV (the psychiatric reference manual), pts may either have the inattentive type, the hyperactive-impulsive type, or the combined type.
Studies show that ADHD may actually result from deficiencies of dopamine in the prefrontal cortex or caudate nucleus, or deficiencies of norepinephrine in the locus ceruleus.
Therefore, treatment attempting to increase these normally activating neurotransmitters should actually correct the problem.

Differential diagnosis
- Absence seizures   - Medication side effect   - Developmental delay
- Street drug effect   - Autism

P **Use a behavior rating scale to make the diagnosis:**
These are usually surveys filled out by the parent, the teacher, and the pt.
Scales include the Connor's, the Barkley, the Achenbach, the SNAP-IV, and the ADHD-T. You should use whichever instrument your institution is most familiar with.
Have the parents return with all three completed forms in 1 to 2 months. If the scores are appropriate, the diagnosis of ADHD can be made and treatment can begin.

Begin treatment with either methylphenidate (Ritalin or Concerta) or an amphetamine (Dexedrine or Adderall).
These are the first-line agents for ADHD.
Concerta is longer-acting than Ritalin but has the same mechanism of action. Start 0.3–0.6 mg/kg/day.
Adderall (the most reliable long-acting medication) and Dexedrine can be given at 0.15–0.3 mg/kg/day.
If your first choice has been ineffective at treating symptoms, you may switch to the other. If the other is also ineffective, second-line therapy is pemoline (Cylert) 1–2 mg/kg/day.

In follow-up visits, monitor for side effects such as irritability, anorexia, nausea, weight loss, insomnia, depression, or growth impairment. Change meds or adjust the dose as needed.

Has the child had shortness of breath caused by cough, wheeze, or chest tightness?

The response to this question can help you diagnose asthma as the problem. Many asthmatics have a chronic nighttime cough, which goes unrecognized. As a result, they are inappropriately treated with cough medicine or antibiotics instead of albuterol and inhaled corticosteroids.

How often do these symptoms occur at night? How often do they occur during the day?

The response helps categorize the asthma (see Table 3).

The categorization is important because it directs treatment.

What makes the asthma symptoms worse or better? What triggers the asthma?

It is important to identify what triggers the child's asthma. Common triggers include:

- Weather changes   - Exercise   - Pollens
- Dust   - Mold   - Cockroaches

If the pt already uses albuterol (or other asthma medications), how often is it used?

If pts report mild symptoms but they use their medicine five nights a week, this could suggest a more severe asthma that is not adequately controlled.

How many times has the child been intubated, hospitalized, or brought to the ER with asthma?

These are important indicators of the severity of the asthma and how aggressively to treat.

Table 3 Asthma Categorizations

Category	Daytime Symptoms	Nighttime Symptoms
Mild Intermittent	$<2 \times$ /wk	$<2 \times$ /mo
Mild Persistent	$>2 \times$ /wk	$>2 \times$ /mo
Moderate Persistent	Daily	Weekly
Severe Persistent	Constant	Frequent

 Look at the pts overall and assess whether they are in respiratory distress based on the following symptoms:

- Unable to speak in full sentences   - Accessory respiratory muscle usage
- Tachypnea   - Tachycardia   - Tripod posture
- Straining facial expression   - Low O_2 saturation

Look closely at the chest wall and abdomen for signs of increased work of breathing.

Sometimes the pt will look fairly comfortable until you take off the shirt and look closely at the chest wall and abdomen to see signs of respiratory distress. These include:

- Subcostal retractions   - Accessory muscle use   - Abdominal breathing

Listen to the chest wall for breath sounds.

Listen for wheezing (a high-pitched sound during expiration), prolonged expiratory phase, and poor air movement. Examine the lungs carefully, auscultating and percussing the lung fields for signs of other lung pathology such as pneumonia.

Always recheck the breath sounds after a breathing treatment.

Often, after a treatment, you may be better able to hear wheezing because there is better air movement.

If breath sounds are unchanged, airways may not be reactive. Other diagnoses should be considered.

 ### Asthma

Asthma is the most common chronic inflammatory disease of the airways. It is a complex pathologic state in which chronic airway inflammation leads to increased mucus production and bronchoconstriction. Bronchoconstriction causes lower airway obstruction, which is intermittent and reversible with bronchodilators.

Differential diagnosis
- Aspirated foreign body
- Heart disease
- Vocal cord dysfunction
- Cystic fibrosis
- Pulmonary infection

Assess severity of disease.
Classify the asthma as Mild Intermittent, Mild Persistent, Moderate Persistent, or Severe Persistent, based on the system noted above.

If the exacerbations occur more than once a day or last several days or are particularly severe (requiring intubation), then the classification should be upgraded.

P ### Explain to the pt how, when, and why to use the asthma medications.
Demonstrate and explain the correct use of the medicine and then observe the pt doing it correctly. Put the spacer on the inhaler and put the other end of the spacer in the mouth. Press down on the inhaler and breathe in slowly for 5 seconds. Hold breath for 10 seconds and then repeat.

Explain the need for spacers.
Ensures that the medicine is small enough particles to reach the lungs.
Without the spacer, much of the medicine deposits in the throat and not the lungs.
Without the spacer, you get more of the side effects and less of the benefits of the medicine.

Explain the difference between relievers and controllers.
Relievers are rescue medicines such as albuterol that are used to stop an exacerbation.
Controllers are medications such as inhaled corticosteroids, leukotriene antagonists, and a long-acting beta-2-agonist that are used daily regardless of how the pt feels.

Prescribe the appropriate medications based on the severity of the asthma.
Mild Intermittent: Albuterol as needed

Mild Persistent: Add a low-dose inhaled corticosteroid twice daily

Moderate Persistent: Increase the dose of corticosteroids to medium, or add a long-acting beta-2-agonist. A leukotriene antagonist or theophylline may substitute for the long-acting beta-2-agonist daily.

Severe Persistent: High-dose inhaled corticosteroids and a long-acting beta-2-agonist twice daily. Add oral corticosteroids as needed. Attempts should be made to reduce corticosteroid dosages at every visit during which symptoms are well controlled.

If the asthma is difficult to control, look for signs of associated diseases and treat them.
The following diseases are often found in association with asthma, and many difficult-to-control asthmatics improve when these specific comorbidities are addressed and treated:
- Allergic rhinitis
- Sinusitis
- Gastric reflux

Does the child have a cough at night or a stuffy nose? If so, how often?
Often this will not be mentioned by the parents and will only come up randomly in one of the routine visits. This question is a good way of screening for allergic rhinitis and other respiratory problems such as asthma. If the parents answer yes, then you should probably follow up with more questions about the actual chronicity and frequency of the problem.

Has the child had his or her tonsils and adenoids removed?
Hypertrophy of the lymphatic tissues that form the Waldeyer ring (including the tonsils and the adenoids) can be responsible for these symptoms.

What other symptoms does the child have?
Runny nose (rhinorrhea)
Red or itchy eyes
Dry, itchy skin
Rashes may imply atopic dermatitis, which is often linked with chronic nasal symptoms.
A chronic cough can be from postnasal drip, asthma, or gastroesophageal reflux disease.

What is the seasonal variation in the child's symptoms?
Discovering a seasonal variation may help uncover an allergy.
- Winter: Cold temperatures can cause tissue swelling. Also, it is the most common time of year for viral infections.
- Spring: Pollen is a very common allergen.
- Summer: Cut grass is another common allergen.
- Fall: Leaf cutting and leaf blowing can lead to these symptoms.

If the child has year-round symptoms, ask about some common household antigens.
- Pets   - Smoking   - Cockroaches   - Dust

Does anyone else in the family have similar problems with allergies, asthma, or snoring?
Family history in the parents, siblings, or other family members can help suggest a diagnosis.

 Examine the ears.
Serous effusion: Clear fluid behind the tympanic membrane suggests swelling, obstructing passage of air through the eustachian tube.

Examine the nose.
Look for edema of the nasal mucosa that is narrowing the passages. Erythema suggests an infection, whereas a boggy, blue color suggests allergy. Also check for polyps (pink, round, fluid-filled structures, protruding down), which suggest that you should start a workup for cystic fibrosis.

Look at the eyes.
Allergic conjunctivitis: Mild erythema or increased vessels in the conjunctiva bilaterally
Allergic shiners: Blue-tinged ring under the eyes

Have the child open his or her mouth in order to view the oropharynx.
Cobblestoning: Oropharyngeal bumps resembling a cobblestone road suggest postnasal drip.
Tonsilar hypertrophy: Tonsils visibly enlarged, touching, or almost touching but not red or purulent in nature. If the tonsil crosses the midline it is 4+, midline is 3+, 1+ is just visible.

Gently press on the child's face over each eyebrow and on each cheekbone.
Pain on this exam suggests the possibility of sinusitis.

Listen to the lungs.
Air should move freely in all areas. Listen for wheezing (a high-pitched noise on expiration); have the pt blow out long and hard to flesh out a wheeze (highly suggestive of asthma).

Examine the skin.
Atopic dermatitis: Dry, scaly, nonerythematous rash, especially in the antecubital fossae

A **Allergic rhinitis**
Allergic rhinitis is a chronic inflammatory disease of the nasal mucosae that affects the sinuses, ears, and throat. It can be exacerbated by a variety of allergens, which are likely to be different in different pts.

Differential diagnosis
Viral upper respiratory infection: Likely to be associated with fever, be less itchy, and be more acute in nature
Nasal foreign body: Unilateral, discrete time of onset, less itchy

Comorbid conditions
As noted above, on exam you may find evidence of:

- Chronic sinusitis	- Tonsillar hypertrophy	- Asthma
- Atopic dermatitis	- Allergic conjunctivitis	- Cystic fibrosis

If you have a difficult time controlling allergic rhinitis, consider that there may be a component of one of these conditions and either investigate the possibility further or just treat empirically.

P **Recommend avoidance of any known allergen.**
If the parent or pt can identify a clear exacerbating factor such as dust, cockroaches, or mold, the best thing is to limit contact with these things. Allergy testing may also be helpful.

Start inhaled nasal steroids, once a day.
These have minimal systemic absorption, so side effects are uncommon. They are highly effective at decreasing the immune response and inflammation, but pts must be aware that they must be used daily, not prn (as needed) for them to work. They do not acutely alleviate symptoms.

Consider a systemic nonsedating antihistamine as the next step in treatment.
Cetirizine, fexofenadine, or loratadine are useful alternatives.

Consider obtaining a sleep study for tonsillar hypertrophy. If (+) for apnea, refer to an ear, nose, and throat (ENT) specialist.
Sleep apnea should not be allowed to continue because it can cause many problems for the pt. The ENT will likely remove the pt's tonsils and adenoids.

If chronic sinusitis is suspected, start amoxicillin 80 mg/kg/day divided into 3 doses for 21 days.
This should be effective treatment, but if symptoms persist, second-line therapy is Augmentin. If that is still not effective, third-line treatment is clindamycin.

Refer to Chronic Cough (p. 44) for a detailed discussion on the treatment of asthma.
Start lubricating eye drops such as Artificial Tears for eye symptoms.
Recommend applying moisturizing creams for suspected atopic dermatitis.
If, after all of the above treatments, your pt does not improve, refer to an allergist.

S **Have parents ever been told the child has a murmur? Are there any symptoms of heart failure, chest pain, exercise intolerance, cyanosis, or syncope?**

Symptoms of heart failure: Tachypnea, poor exercise tolerance, sweating with feeds, poor weight gain, pallor, periorbital edema, cool extremities.

If there is chest pain, ask specifically about location, radiation, frequency, duration, exacerbating or relieving factors, palpitations, dizziness, syncope.

If cyanosis is intermittent, ask about precipitating factors such as breath-holding or eating.

If there is exercise intolerance, ask about normal activity, comparison with peers, relation to fatigue.

For pts with syncope, see Syncope p. 64.

Has the child had rheumatic fever (RF) or any of its signs or symptoms?

The Jones major criteria for RF (a good mnemonic is J ♥NES):
- *Joints* (arthritis)   - ♥ (carditis)   - *N*odes
- *E*rythema marginatum   - *S*ydenham chorea

Were any drugs or medications taken during pregnancy (most likely heart lesion in parentheses)?

Hydantoin (ventricular septal defect [VSD], pulmonary stenosis, aortic stenosis [AS], patent ductus arteriosus [PDA], coarctation)

Valproate (atrial septal defect [ASD], VSD)

Lithium (Ebstein anomaly)

Alcohol (ASD, PDA, VSD, ToF)

Retinoic acid (aortic and conotruncal abnormalities)

Are there any congenital abnormalities or a family history of heart disease?

Trisomy 13, 18, and 21 (VSD)

DiGeorge (ToF, truncus arteriosus)

Williams (supravalvular aortic stenosis, peripheral pulmonary stenosis)

Turner (coarctation, bicuspid aortic valve)

Ehlers-Danlos (mitral valve prolapse [MVP], tricuspid valve prolapse, aortic dilation)

Marfan (MVP, aortic dilation/dissection)

Family history of congenital heart disease, sudden death or myocardial infarction (MI) in <50-yr-old, diabetes mellitus, or hypertension

O **Look at the general appearance.**

Consider syndromes such as VACTERL, DiGeorge, Turner, Williams, and Marfan.

Is there a murmur and, if so, is it systolic or diastolic?

To assess whether a murmur is systolic or diastolic, listen very carefully for S_1 and S_2. S_1 should coincide with the pulse and S_2 should split with inspiration. Systole comes after S_1, diastole after S_2.

Where is the murmur best heard?

Aortic sounds: 2nd intercostal space, right upper sternal border

Pulmonic sounds: 2nd intercostal space, left upper sternal border

Tricuspid sounds, VSD: 4th intercostal space, left lower sternal border

Mitral sounds: 4th to 5th intercostal space, midclavicular line with axillary radiation

What does the murmur sound like?

In general, stenosis murmurs are crescendo-decrescendo, and regurgitant murmurs have a uniform sound, with onset coinciding with the valve closure.

What is the grade of the murmur?

Grade I (Very hard to hear), II (Easy to hear), III (Loud/no thrill), IV (Loud/thrill), V (Loud with stethoscope near chest), VI (No stethoscope needed)

After examining the heart, perform a focused PE.

Feel for a hyperdynamic or displaced precordium, thrills, pulses, and organomegaly.
Listen carefully to the lungs for rales or wheezes.
Check for clubbing, cyanosis, retractions, and chest surgery scars.

Heart murmur

Murmurs and bruits, which can be auscultated and sometimes palpated, are created
whenever there is turbulent blood flow. The more turbulent the flow, the louder a
murmur.

Differential diagnosis

Innocent murmurs:

- *Still's murmur:* By far the most common. A systolic vibratory or twanging sound
  that can be heard at the left lower sternal border and over the mitral valve. Most
  common in children 4 to 6 yrs old but can be any age.
- *Venous hum:* A continuous murmur (not associated with heart sounds) that can
  only be heard in the sitting-up position. Usually heard just under the clavicles
  bilaterally, it is the sound of venous blood returning from the head to the heart. It
  sounds like a cascading waterfall.
- *Flow murmur:* Can be aortic or pulmonic, occasionally Grade III but usually less,
  they are whispering midsystolic sounds. They do not sound harsh like stenosis
  murmurs.
- *Mammary soufflé:* The pulsing sound of increased arterial blood flow to the
  breast, it only occurs in pregnant women.

If the murmur is not one of these, it is likely pathologic. The most common include:

- *Ventricular septal defect (VSD):* A regurgitant murmur at the left lower sternal
  border. It may last throughout systole or may terminate midsystole if the defect
  closes as the septum contracts. The murmur is louder as the defect becomes
  smaller.
- *Aortic stenosis (AS):* A loud, harsh systolic murmur, soft at the end of S_1, loud in
  midsystole, and soft before S_2 over the aortic area. Note that in the case of
  congenital bicuspid aortic valve, this murmur is associated with an early systolic
  click over the mitral valve area.
- *Patent ductus arteriosus (PDA):* Usually a continuous murmur with a "washing
  machine"–type quality. It is best heard in the left midclavicular line at the second
  intercostal space.
- *Mitral stenosis:* Rarely occurs in pts who have not had rheumatic fever, it presents
  as a low-pitched, diastolic rumble after an opening snap that radiates to the left
  axilla.
- *Mitral valve prolapse (MVP):* No sound is heard after S_1 and then a midsystolic
  click or pop can be heard, followed by a soft blowing sound over the mitral area,
  which lasts until S_2. It is more common in women and pts with Marfan's
  syndrome.
- *Atrial septal defect (ASD):* Doesn't cause a murmur per se, but it causes a fixed
  split to the S_2 (which should normally only be split during inspiration) and, in
  later years, can mimic tricuspid stenosis as increased right-sided blood volume
  pours over a size-restricted tricuspid valve.

Get an echocardiogram, ECG, chest x-ray, and consult cardiology if a pathologic murmur is suspected.

All of the above pathologic murmurs can cause serious problems for the pt in the
future. ECG and chest x-ray will be helpful, but the echocardiogram will definitively
characterize the lesion and the cardiologist will have to evaluate it.

S **What are the symptoms of constipation in this pt?**

Constipation occurs when the lower colon does not completely evacuate. Symptoms include:

- Involuntary soiling (encopresis)	- Pain with defecation
- Decreasing stool frequency	- Hard stools

Occasional painful defecation and decreased stool frequency alone do not constitute constipation. A child who has only two stools per week is not constipated if these stools are large and soft, and the child is fully evacuated when finished.

At what age did the child become constipated?

Functional constipation: Onset is with a transition in feeding or stooling pattern:

- Breast milk to formula	- Baby food to table food	-Starting cow's milk
- New toilets (preschool)	- Toilet training	

Hirschsprung disease: Onset is at birth. Usually the child was kept in the hospital for a delayed first bowel movement.

Does the child soil his or her underwear?

Encopresis (fecal incontinence) represents severe constipation. The colon continues to absorb water from the impacted or retained stool. Soon a large, dry mass plugs up the distal colon and rectum. New liquid stool leaks around the hard mass and is deposited in the underwear.

What are the stools like?

History of small, hard ball–like stools implies incomplete evacuation of any kind. Rare passage of large, voluminous stools indicates functional stool retention. Pencil-thin stools and a lack of encopresis are more indicative of Hirschsprung's.

Is there a family history of constipation or of a constipating disease?

- Hirschsprung's	- Cystic fibrosis	- Hypothyroidism
- Neurofibromatosis	- Myopathies	

O **Check the growth curves for height and weight.**

Failure to grow correctly is a red flag for the aforementioned genetic or metabolic diseases.

Perform a complete neurologic exam, including normal sensation of the perineum.

An occult myelomeningocele (a disorder where a portion of the spinal cord protrudes through a partially fused spine) can present with mild lower extremity weakness or no more than saddle anesthesia and constipation with encopresis.

Examine the abdomen.

Listen for normal bowel sounds.

Palpate the abdomen. Make sure that it is soft and feel for balls of retained stool. Mild tenderness diffusely is consistent with chronic constipation.

Examine the anus externally.

Look for fissures or signs of local infection that may produce pain on defecation.

A rectal exam is necessary if you have reason to suspect Hirschsprung's.

Use a lubricated, gloved finger. A normal anal canal will be tight initially, but will relax within moments. A canal that remains tight should lead you to consider Hirschsprung's or some other cause of distal rectal obstruction.

A plain x-ray of the abdomen may be necessary if the History and PE are inconclusive.
Impacted stool will be very clear on KUB.

If you continue to suspect Hirschsprung's, send the pt for a barium enema.
The rectum should be the largest structure; in Hirschsprung's, it is smaller than the sigmoid.

A Constipation

Infantile rectal confusion: Infants cannot voluntarily retain stool, but they can develop an inability to coordinate their Valsalva maneuver with pelvic floor relaxation.

Stool holding or functional constipation (most common): Begins when the child is faced with a situation when he or she feels the urge to defecate, but for some reason wishes to prevent it. This causes little problem in the short-term, but over long periods, the distal colon and rectum begin to become distended. The child resists passing the large, hard stool for as long as possible because of the expected pain. When the stool passes, their expectations are fulfilled. For a few days their symptoms are relieved, but the cycle continues.

Hirschsprung's disease: A defect of the rectum beginning at the anus involving a variable distance of rectum and even colon. The involved large bowel fails to develop normal innervation, so when stool arrives it fails to dilate. The proximal normal bowel distends until it is noticed and corrected surgically.

Differential diagnosis
Lack of stool: Infantile botulism, irritable bowel syndrome, intestinal atresia/stenosis
Encopresis: Crohn's disease, ulcerative colitis, bloody diarrhea (colitis), cystic fibrosis, malabsorptive syndromes
Pain on defecation: Rectal fissures/fistulas, herpes
Blood in stool: Colitis, fissure/hemorrhoids, rarely cancer

P Educate the parents regarding the threefold treatment of functional constipation.
Increased dietary fiber is ineffective until muscle tone is restored. Treatment failure is common and usually results from weaning medications too quickly. Even with proper treatment, up to 50% recur.

Start with total evacuation, the first phase of treatment.
Mineral oil followed by enemas. Polyethylene glycol orally for 2 to 5 days.

Next recommend diet changes, behavior modification, and medications to maintain evacuation.
Place pt on a low-dairy, low-fiber diet and give oral mineral oil, milk of magnesia, or lactulose.
Encourage child to use the toilet with positive rewards and a daily star chart.

If evacuation is sustained after 3 to 12 months, slowly wean the medication.
Decrease by one dose each month until the medication is stopped.
May use a bisacodyl suppository if the child goes 3 days without stooling.

If the barium enema indicates Hirschsprung's, refer to a surgeon for a biopsy looking for aganglionic bowel.

S **Has the child always been small or has he or she just recently stopped growing?**
A child who has always been small may have genetic short stature. The parents may not be very tall, or the child may have a genetic syndrome.

Was the child small at birth?
A child with intrauterine growth restriction may have a genetic reason to be small.

What are the parents' expectations for the child's height?
Occasionally, short parents have unrealistic expectations of their child's height.

Obtain the height of both parents and whether either had a delayed growth spurt
Using this information a mid-parental height can be calculated to see if the family has delayed growth.

Does the child have any chronic illnesses that the parents know of?
All of the following can cause short stature:

- Inflammatory bowel disease	- Renal disease	- Congenital heart disease
- Chronic anemias	- Diabetes	- Liver disease
- Celiac disease	- Cystic fibrosis	-Asthma
- Treatment with steroids		

How is the child eating?
Malnutrition can be a cause of short stature (e.g., a picky eater who consumes no protein).

O **Plot the child's growth on a standardized growth chart.**
The child's height may fall within the normal range for age.
It is very common for the parent to think that the child is short when he or she is actually normal.
If the child is below the 5th percentile for height, it is important to recheck to make sure that the measurement was done accurately.
- Three heights should be measured with a stadiometer and then averaged.
- Make sure the child has his or her head, shoulders, and bottom against the wall.
If this is not the pt's first visit to the clinic, there should be other data available on the growth chart. Check a growth velocity. Normal growth is as follows:
- Toddlers grow 7.5 cm to 13 cm in the second year of life.
- From 3 yrs to puberty, children should grow at about 5 cm to 6.5 cm per year.
- Adolescents have a variable growth rate, but increased growth follows the onset of puberty. Girls generally begin puberty at age 10 yrs, whereas boys start later, at about age 12.5 years. If a girl reaches age 13 or a boy 15 with no signs of puberty, this should be investigated.
A child who is below the 5th percentile but has normal growth velocity is probably normal.
If the growth velocity is less than normal, it should be worked up.

Plot a mid-parental height on the growth chart.
For girls it is [(the father's height − 13 cm) + the mother's height]/2.
For boys it is [(the mother's height + 13 cm) + the father's height]/2.
A child's target height is the mid-parental height ± two standard deviations (about 10 cm).

Therefore, a child's current percentile spot should track to the mid-parental height
± 10 cm. If it does, then the child's height is appropriate, even if the child is less than
the 5th percentile.

Now plot the child's weight.
Weight should track to a similar percentile as height.
If the child is obese compared with the current height, and the child is tracking to
below the mid-parental height, consider an endocrinopathy such as:
   - Hypothyroidism   - Cushing's syndrome   - Growth hormone deficiency
If the child's weight percentile is below where the height is plotted, and the child is
tracking to below the mid-parental height, consider a chronic disease such as:
   - Renal failure   - Cystic fibrosis
   - Celiac disease   - Inflammatory bowel disease

Perform a generalized PE, looking for signs of chronic disease.
A child with hypothyroidism may have coarse skin, hair loss, and eyebrow thinning.
Cushing's syndrome may present with centripetal obesity, muscle wasting, and striae.
Hepatosplenomegaly and jaundice are consistent with chronic liver disease.
Abnormal features may indicate a genetic or chromosomal anomaly. Webbed neck,
shield chest, and widely spaced nipples may indicate Noonan or Turner syndromes.

**If the pt does not track to near the mid-parental height, check a CBC,
an erythrocyte sedimentation rate (ESR), a Chem 7, a thyroid-
stimulating hormone, and order a radiographic bone age.**
These labs will help you rapidly rule out renal failure, inflammatory disorders (if the
ESR is normal), and hypothyroidism.

A **Familial Short Stature versus Constitutional Growth Delay**
Familial short stature: The pt is less than 5th percentile for height, has a normal growth
velocity, and tracks to the appropriate mid-parental height. The pt is genetically short.
Constitutional growth delay: These pts are less than 5th percentile, have a normal growth
velocity, and a delayed bone age. Labs are normal. The pt will be a "late-bloomer,"
have a growth spurt later on, and catch up to where he or she needs to be.

**Differential diagnosis of abnormal growth velocity and delayed bone
age**
   - Renal disease   - GI disease   - Hypothyroidism
   - Cushing's syndrome   - Genetic syndrome   - Growth hormone deficiency
   - Cerebral palsy   - Cystic fibrosis   - Any chronic condition

Abnormal growth velocity with advanced bone age
Precocious puberty

P **If the child has familial short stature or constitutional growth delay,
give reassurance.**
In the case of constitutional growth delay, the child will grow normally and will achieve
the expected mid-parental height. In the case of familial short stature, the child will
not be tall, but is appropriate. No treatment is needed.

**For suspected endocrinopathies or chronic diseases, refer to an
endocrinologist for possible growth hormone therapy.**

S **How often does the child have nosebleeds?**
Chronicity may imply an ongoing problem such as:
- Nose-picking   - Dry environment
- Telangiectasia   - Bleeding diathesis

How long do the nosebleeds last?
If the nosebleed is treated appropriately, it should not last more than a few minutes.

What is the child doing to stop the bleeding when it occurs?
Stopping a nosebleed requires tight pressure applied just anterior to the bony part of
the nose for about 2 to 5 minutes without checking to see if it is still bleeding.
If the child is holding the pressure up on the bone instead of in front of it or leaning
over a bowl with ice on the forehead and not holding the nose, bleeding may last
longer than expected.

Which side of the nose bleeds?
Nosebleeds tend to occur from only one nostril.
When the pt has bleeding from both nostrils at once, this should make you concerned
regarding a problem with clotting (see Easy Bruising or Mucosal Bleeding p. 88).

Ask the child "Which finger do you use to pick your nose?"
Trauma from nose-picking is far and away the most common reason for recurrent
nosebleeds, and this question has a way of surprising the answer out of children.

**Does the child have cold symptoms such as cough, runny nose, stuffy
nose, etc.?**
Although it would be rare for the parents to leave this information out of the History,
upper respiratory infections are associated with nosebleeds.
Nasal congestion may lead to the parent using a topical decongestant spray. These tend
to irritate the nasal mucosa and may cause bleeding.

Is the child coughing up or spitting up blood?
This is a symptom of inappropriate therapy. It is often worrisome for the parents, who
will usually bring it up on their own.
Implies the head is being held back to stop the bleeding and blood is dripping into the
throat.

**Does the child put foreign bodies (tissue, marbles, etc.) in his or her
nose?**
Foreign bodies can cause nosebleeds from irritation and erosion of the mucosa.

O **Is the child actively bleeding at this time?**
If the child is actively bleeding, stop the bleeding using the technique described above.

How does the child appear?
Other than slightly frightened over the nosebleed, the child should appear well with a
normal energy level and entirely interactive with the parent and you. Check for any
pallor or jaundice.

Using an otoscope with a speculum, examine the inside of the nose.
If the child has been bleeding recently, you may see dried blood in one nare.
The mucosa should appear pink and healthy.
Make note of any clusters of capillaries (telangiectasias) on the mucosa.
Mucosa that has been exposed to chronic decongestant use may appear red and
swollen, leaving little room for the passage of air.

Blue, boggy mucosa may be irritated because of allergies.

If you live in a dry climate, or it has been dry recently, the mucosa may appear dry.

A foreign body should be apparent if it is present.

In an older child or adolescent, rarely the mucosa will appear black. This may be a sign of a necrotizing lesion. The Differential diagnosis is small:

- Cocaine usage can cause necrosis of the septum and nosebleeds.
- In diabetics or neutropenics, a fungal infection called *Mucor* can have this appearance. It is an emergency referral to otolaryngology (ENT).
- Wegener's granulomatosis

Complete a rapid PE.

A blowing heart murmur or an S_3 may represent high-output heart failure secondary to extreme blood loss or anemia.

Note any hepatosplenomegaly or other abdominal masses.

A petechial rash (small red spots that do not blanch when you press on them) represents bleeding under the skin. Together with nosebleeds, this is a sure sign that the child has a bleeding diathesis such as idiopathic thrombocytopenic purpura (ITP).

Blood dripping down into the oropharynx represents a posterior nasal cavity bleed.

A ### Epistaxis (nosebleed)

Epistaxis is commonly associated with a set of blood vessels known as Kiesselbach's plexus. This plexus may bleed spontaneously, although picking is the most likely cause.

Differential diagnosis

Bleeding diathesis: von Willebrand's disease, hemophilia, leukemia, ITP

Other processes: Wegener's granulomatosis, nasal steroids, mucormycosis, vitamin C deficiency, vitamin K deficiency, taking aspirin, being on heparin, nasal cocaine

P ### First, stop the bleeding as indicated above. Educate the parents on how to do the same.

Parental education should also include the benign nature of the disease and that nose-picking may be the cause. Parents also need to understand that nasal decongestants cannot be used chronically without serious side effects on the nasal mucosa.

If bleeding cannot be stopped, or there is reason to suspect a bleeding disorder, check a CBC with differential, PT, PTT, and a chem panel.

This should help rule in or rule out a chronic disease.

If the bleeding still cannot be stopped, call ENT for packing or cautery.

Remember that adolescent males may have a benign tumor of the sinuses called an angiofibroma. It may cause recurrent bleeding and will require ENT evaluation as well.

S **What is the pt doing about his or her acne?**
This is a way of bringing up the topic. Many times, acne is not the chief complaint. It will not even be mentioned as a problem until you bring it up, but when you do, you will usually see the pt respond with relief and interest that you addressed the issue.
It is also important to know what medications have been used in the past or are currently being used to attempt to treat the acne so therapy can be tailored appropriately.

What medications are being used?
It is important to obtain a drug history. Those medications for other conditions that may worsen acne include:

- Corticosteroids	- Lithium	- Isoniazid
- Rifampin	- Hydantoin	

Oral contraceptive pills may worsen or improve acne.

What hair or cosmetic products are being used?
Makeup with lanolin or oil or any grease used in the hair can worsen acne.

How many times a day does the pt wash his or her face?
It is important that the pt understand that frequent washing with harsh soaps can actually make acne worse. Adolescents should only wash once or twice a day with a mild soap.

What type of activities is the pt involved in at school or after school?
Activities such as football, with helmets, shoulder pads, etc., can worsen acne.
If the teen is involved in working out at the gym, you may want to ask if he or she is using anabolic steroids. These are certain to increase acne.

When was the pt's last menstrual period, and have they been regular?
Oligomenorrhea may suggest other comorbid conditions that worsen acne (see below). However, it is worth noting that adolescents in the first two years of their menstrual cycle commonly have irregular and infrequent periods.

Ask if the pt is sexually active.
Some of the acne medications, including isotretinoin (Accutane) and tetracycline can be extremely teratogenic. Using two forms of contraception simultaneously is advised.

O **Observe the lesions and describe what you see.**
Acne lesions can be broken down into three groups:
- *Obstructive lesions:* Comedones are small, white (closed comedones) or black (open comedones) papules that may or may not be surrounded by an area of erythema. These are the "whiteheads" and "blackheads," respectively.
- *Inflammatory lesions:* Erythematous papules, pustules, or nodules. Pts with nodules are more likely to develop cysts and scars, so they should be treated aggressively.
- *Cysts and scars:* Cysts are nodular lesions without overlying erythema, and scars have the appearance of pits. These are often irreversible changes, so these pts should be treated aggressively.

Carefully examine the face, chest, and back and be careful to document the numbers of each type of acne lesion in each area so an assessment of improvement can be made at the next visit.

A

Acne (see below for classification)
Acne occurs when the sebaceous glands that make the oil that coats the skin become clogged. This becomes extremely common with the hormonal changes seen in adolescence. Open comedones are black because environmental dirt colors them. Inflammatory lesions have become infected with *P. acnes*, an anaerobic organism that is ubiquitous on the skin.

Differential diagnosis
Acne has a fairly typical appearance that is not usually confused with other entities, but you should consider the following:
- Tuberous sclerosis syndrome   - Polycystic ovarian disease
- Congenital adrenal hyperplasia   - Cushing's syndrome
- Obesity   - Pregnancy

You may also see acne-like lesions in babies. This is neonatal acne or neonatal pustular melanosis, neither of which requires treatment.

Consider activities or products that may be contributing to the acne.
Activities like football or working in greasy environments like fast-food restaurants can exacerbate acne and, in severe cases with nodules or scaring, pts should consider avoiding these activities.

Hair care products and make-up are good examples of things that can be changed or removed from the daily routine to improve the acne.

Assess the severity of the acne (Table 4).
The more lesions and locations and the more scars or nodules that are seen, the more aggressively you should treat the acne.

Table 4 Acne Classification

Type of Acne	Total Lesions	Comedones	Inflammatory	Cysts
Mild	<30	<20	<15	0
Moderate	30–125	20–100	15–50	<5
Severe	>125	>100	>50	>5

P

Recommend washing with gentle soap at most twice a day.
Clarify that acne is not improved and can actually be made worse with frequent washing.

Point out that the make-up or hair products they are using may be worsening their acne.

For mild acne, start with 5% benzoyl peroxide gel once a day.
For pts with moderate acne, start with 5% benzoyl peroxide gel plus (depending on type):
For comedonal acne: Tretinoin 0.025% cream nightly (to avoid the side effect of sun sensitivity)
For inflammatory acne: Clindamycin 1% cream twice a day

For pts with severe acne, use benzoyl peroxide, tretinoin, and oral erythromycin or tetracycline.
Consider referral to dermatology to limit or prevent permanent scar formation.
The dermatologist may wish to start the pt on Accutane.

IV
Pediatric Emergency Room

S **Is there a constellation of symptoms suggestive of anaphylaxis?**
Neuro: Feelings of doom, mouth tingling, tightness in the chest
Resp: Shortness of breath
CV: Dizziness, palpitations
FEN/GI: Stomach pain, nausea/vomiting, diarrhea
Ob/Gyn: Menstrual cramping
Derm: Hives, itching

Ask about previous episodes or history of allergies or anaphylaxis.
A history of allergic reactions or anaphylaxis in the past to things such as peanuts, seafood, antibiotics, or insect stings will increase your clinical suspicion.

Ask specifically about exposure to medicines, food, and insects or recent exercise.
Drugs: Sulfonamides, penicillins, antiepileptics
Foods: Peanuts, tree nuts, crustaceans
Stings: Hymenoptera venom
Other less common but well-known causes of anaphylaxis include latex, vaccines, hormones, aspirin, and exercise.
  • Latex allergies commonly cross-react with stone fruits such as avocado, plum, peach, or cherry.

What was the time course of the reaction?
Most anaphylaxis occurs within 30 minutes of exposure (although it can be longer with ingestions), and in some cases there may be a recurrence 1 to 8 hrs later. The more rapidly the anaphylaxis occurs and progresses, the more likely the reaction is to be severe and life threatening.

O **Examine the pt.**
Vital signs: Hypotension and tachycardia are extremely common. Tachypnea would also be expected.
Neuro: The pt may have altered mental status, a late sign of shock.
Oropharynx: Tongue and pharyngeal swelling (causing muffling of the voice) can both occur as hallmark symptoms of angioedema.
Lungs: Wheeze and stridor are both common in anaphylaxis.
Skin: Sweating is common, but the most common finding is of urticaria (erythematous, raised lesions on the skin that may change location), commonly known as hives. The pt may be scratching them.
  • Urticaria and angioedema are the most common symptoms of anaphylaxis (>90%).
  • The next most common manifestations are respiratory difficulty, then dizziness, syncope, and GI symptoms.

Labs
β-tryptase level can be drawn to confirm the diagnosis in retrospect. A level above 10 ng/mL indicates mast cell activation.

A **Anaphylaxis or, at its worst, anaphylactic shock**
Anaphylaxis occurs when the immune system is exposed to an allergen, recognized by an immunoglobulin E (IgE) antibody bound to the surface of a mast cell. If the allergen is present in sufficient number as to cause cross-linking of IgE on the mast cell surface, the mast cell is stimulated to degranulate. Its inflammatory cytokines,

especially histamine, induce multiple changes, including massive vasodilation and capillary leak.

Differential diagnosis

- Hypovolemic shock   - Septic shock   - Cardiogenic shock
- Panic disorder   - Foreign body aspiration   - Acute intoxication
- Pulmonary embolus   - Seizure   - Vasovagal reaction

- Vasovagal reaction will present with bradycardia, whereas anaphylaxis presents with tachycardia.
- Rarely will any of the above diagnoses be concurrent with urticaria.

P **Quickly check responsiveness, assess ABCs, and then place an oxygen delivery system (nasal cannula, or face mask), secure an IV, and attach a monitor.**

Shock is a medical emergency and should be dealt with as such. Assessing the ABCs is always a good place to start.

Place the pt supine with the feet higher than the head.
This will allow for adequate blood return to the heart (and thus to the brain) by gravity.

Administer epinephrine, 1:1000 (1 mg/mL) at a dose of 0.01 mL/kg (max 0.3 mL in children and 0.5 mL in adults). Repeat Epi as needed every 15 minutes.
The number-one drug for treating anaphylaxis is epinephrine.
It can be given intravenously or via an intraosseous line. If no access has been secured, it can even be given down the endotracheal tube.

Consider endotracheal intubation if necessary for laryngeal edema or respiratory failure.
Signs of this include worsening stridor or hypoxia over time.

If hypotensive, give boluses of NS 10–20 cc/kg and consider pressors such as dopamine.
This may be necessary to counteract the massive vasodilation.

If source is insect bite, consider placing tourniquet above reaction site. Be sure to release the tourniquet about every 3 minutes.
This will prevent further circulation of the toxin.

Also administer:
Diphenhydramine **or** hydroxyzine (H_1 blocker)
Famotidine, ranitidine, **or** cimetidine (H_2 blocker)
Albuterol
Hydrocortisone

If the pt is not improving on these medications or has required intubation, admit to the Pediatric Intensive Care Unit. Otherwise, give discharge instructions and a prescription for a home epinephrine delivery system.
Tell the pt to avoid the allergen and to return to the ER if the symptoms recur.
Educate on the proper use and storage of home epinephrine.

If this is a recurrent event, and the allergen is unknown, refer to an allergist for testing.

S **When did the seizure start?**
Status epilepticus is defined as more than 30 minutes of continuous seizure activity or two or more sequential seizures without full recovery of consciousness between seizures.
The longer the seizure lasts, the more refractory it becomes to treatment.
Treat seizures lasting longer than 10 minutes as if they are status epilepticus.

What did the seizure look like?
Generalized tonic-clonic seizures: Characterized by whole body stiffening then shaking
Partial seizures: Demonstrate one specific body part twitching or shaking
Absence seizures: Brief spells of staring

What was the child doing before the seizure started?
More specifically, was there head trauma, prolonged fast, or a new medicine before the seizure?

Has the child had a seizure before?
A first-time seizure or new seizure pattern prompts more of an investigation (head CT scan or MRI and EEG) than another seizure in a pt with a known seizure disorder.

Does the child have a known brain disorder?
Cerebral palsy, autism, and many genetic lesions are associated with seizure. Even if the child has never had a seizure before, these conditions would suggest the onset of a seizure disorder.

Did the child have a fever?
If seizure occurs at the time of a fever, consider two things: meningitis and febrile seizure.

 Is the pt stable?
Look at the pulse oximeter and vital signs. If they are not stable, go back to the ABCs (i.e., airway, breathing, circulation) of pediatric advanced life support and consider intubation if a gag reflex is absent.

Is the pt still having a seizure?
Neuro exam: Responsiveness, pupillary reaction, reflexes, posture, tone
Seizure stopped: Responsive and verbally follows commands (if age appropriate)
Seizure ongoing: Tachycardia, eye deviation, increased tone, and/or clonic movements

If febrile and between the ages of 6 months and 6 yrs, look for a source of infection.
This especially pertains to the ears, throat, and urine. Identifying a source of fever may save this child from having a lumbar puncture if you suspect febrile seizure.

Check some stat labs to rule out some of the common/easily modifiable causes of seizures.
Glucose: Hypoglycemia can precipitate a seizure. May check quickly by fingerstick.
Electrolytes: If the seizure is ongoing. Hypo/hypernatremia can both cause seizures.
Consider a blood and urine toxicology screen (see Chemical Ingestions p. 82).
Antiepileptic medication levels: Check for low levels, indicating a need for either increased dose or increased adherence to therapy.

Seizure
Seizures represent massive neuronal discharge in the brain, producing physical symptoms.

Differential diagnosis
Generalized tonic clonic (GTC) or grand mal: Stiffening, then shaking of the entire body.
Absence (petit mal): Generalized seizure with loss of consciousness (LOC). Subtle movements (blinking/lip-smacking). Lasts seconds. EEG shows 3-Hz spike and wave pattern.
Complex partial: Starts with abnormal movements restricted to one part of the body. Consciousness is lost. Commonly, secondary generalization occurs.
Simple partial: This rare seizure type involves abnormal movements of only one body part. The "simple" designates the fact that there is no LOC.
West syndrome (infantile spasm) (poor prognosis): Neurodegenerative disorder that presents at about 3 to 6 months of age with a unique seizure where the infant bends at the waist and throws arms out to the sides.

Febrile seizure versus meningitis
Febrile seizures: Are usually GTC and last <15 minutes. Postictal period tends to be short and mild. Rarely occur in children before 6 months of age and never after 6 yrs. They are completely benign (no damage to the brain) and are extremely unlikely to recur.
Meningitis: If the seizure was focal, lasted >15 minutes, the pt had >1 seizure, is <6 months or >6 yrs, or is obtunded, then rule out meningitis. Check CT, LP, and admission for observation.
For pts with known seizure disorder, fever lowers the seizure threshold.

P **If there is no resolution within 10 minutes, give IV lorazepam 0.1 mg/kg or rectal diazepam 0.4 mg/kg. Repeat lorazepam if there is no resolution in 5 minutes.**
Benzodiazepines are central nervous system (CNS) depressants that are safe and effective at stopping seizures.

If the seizure continues, give phosphenytoin 20 phenytoin equivalents/kg IV q 15 minutes up to two times. Then begin a maintenance dose of 2 mg/kg q 12 hours if the seizure stops.
Phenytoin (Dilantin) stabilizes sodium channels and is highly effective at stopping a seizure. Phosphenytoin is a preparation that runs faster in an IV and causes less local tissue damage.

If the seizure continues, intubate and give phenobarbital 20 mg/kg loading dose and then 5 mg/kg/dose q 15 minutes until seizure controlled.
Barbiturates, like benzodiazepines, are effective CNS depressants.

Consider a Versed or propofol drip for further active seizure activity.

Admit:
Intubated pts who are still having a seizure to the ICU.
New-onset seizures (unless they are febrile or absence) for workup.
All suspected meningitides for treatment.

Discharge:
Suspected febrile seizure pts home with parental reassurance.
Pts with known seizure disorders whose seizures have stopped. Be sure to redose their medications.
Suspected absence seizures with an outpatient EEG and neurology clinic follow-up.

S **Have the parent and child (if old enough) and any witnesses available describe the event.**

Often the parent will tell you that the child appeared pale, diaphoretic, and nonresponsive.

Rarely, you will hear of involuntary, "seizure-like" movements and urinary incontinence. This history does not necessarily indicate a seizure.

Pt's symptomatic prodrome often includes:
- Lightheadedness   - Darkening visual field   - Auditory changes
- Headache   - Nausea

Unconsciousness should not last more than a minute or two.

What was the child doing before loss of consciousness (LOC)?

Syncope during exercise: Represents cardiac pathology until proven otherwise.

Vasovagal reaction: Caused by activities that increase intrathoracic pressure, such as coughing, urinating, defecating, and even strong emotions such as fear or surprise.

Prolonged upright posture: Especially in a warm environment with knees locked, can lead to blood pooling in the lower extremities and poor venous return.

Breath holding: A benign syncope in infants and toddlers in which the child gets so worked up during a temper tantrum that he or she does not breathe.

Hyperventilation: Reduces serum carbon dioxide levels. When this happens, cerebral blood flow decreases and unconsciousness may ensue.

Has this ever occurred before?

Benign reflex syncope (vasovagal response) often recurs for 1 to 2 yrs and then resolves.
History of previous syncope with exercise raises suspicion of cardiac disease.

Ask about other possible symptoms of cardiac syncope:

Palpitations or chest pains before LOC

Lack of warning signs, especially if there was an injury with the associated fall (a pt with a vasovagal response is likely to gently slump to the ground or try to lie down).

Has the pt had a recent history of increasing fatigue or decreasing exercise tolerance?

This may be another sign of a worsening cardiac lesion.

Is there a family history of syncope, early-unexplained death, or any other heart problem?

All of these should once again prompt a cardiac evaluation.

O **Begin by checking the pt's vital signs.**

Tachyarrhythmias and bradycardia can both be causes of syncope.

Carefully check orthostatic blood pressure.

Have the pt lay supine for 2 minutes. Record the heart rate and BP.
Have the pt sit up for 3 minutes. Record the heart rate and BP again.
Have the pt stand for 5 minutes. This gives the final heart rate and BP.
If the heart rate increases by more than 15 bpm or the systolic blood pressure drops by more than 20 mm Hg on any change of position or between lying down and standing, the pt is said to be orthostatic.
This may indicate a low circulating blood volume or that the autonomic nervous system is not compensating well for postural changes.

Perform a thorough cardiac exam and auscultate in both the supine and upright positions.

Record all murmurs and rhythm irregularities. Checking in both positions is important because some pathologic murmurs can be positional. Hypertrophic obstructive cardiomyopathy (HOCM) is a common cause of LOC and sudden cardiac death in these pts. The murmur is systolic and harsh and decreases with passive leg raise.

Obtain an ECG.

Arrhythmias: Ventricular tachycardia, supraventricular tachycardia, heart block
Electrical disturbances:

- *Wolff-Parkinson-White (WPW) anomaly:* An accessory pathway carries electrical signals around the AV node. Shortened PR interval and slurred QRS upstroke (delta wave).
- *Prolonged QT syndrome:* Characterized by a QT interval corrected for rate (QTc) greater than 450 ms. At that rate, a new QRS complex can occur before T wave repolarization has finished, causing an R on T phenomenon, and ventricular tachycardia can result.

A   **Benign Reflex Syncope (a.k.a. Vasovagal Response)**

Pt develops an increased vagal tone, causing bradycardia and hypotension, which resolves when the pt is horizontal and gravity allows redistribution of blood to the brain.

Must rule out neurologic and cardiac causes to make this diagnosis.

Although up to one-quarter of the pediatric population (including adolescents) will develop syncope at some point in their lives, significant pathology is found in <10% of pts.

Differential diagnosis

Breath-holding spell: Benign LOC usually occurs in a crying infant/toddler.
ALTE: See Infant Who Stops Breathing or Changes Color p. 68.
Seizures: Involuntarily shaking, convulsion, staring, blinking, or lip-smacking. May not have a prodrome. Lightheadedness and slumping to the ground are uncommon. Pts tend to have minor injuries, including tongue biting. Injury is more common in seizure than syncope.
Cardiac abnormality: WPW, HOCM, long QT syndrome, anomalous coronary artery

P   **If you suspect a cardiac cause, admit the pt and obtain an echocardiogram and cardiology consult.**

Because of risk of sudden death, monitor the pt until pathology is ruled out or corrected.

For vasovagal responses, encourage increased hydration and increased dietary salt intake.

Explain that the child is normal, and although this may recur, it is entirely benign.

If benign syncope is recurrent, you may refer your pt for a tilt-table test.

In this test, the pt is strapped to a table that is rotated to a 90-degree position and held there for 10 to 60 minutes. This may aid in the diagnosis of an etiology for recurrent syncope.

S **Does the child have a history of asthma?**
Previously diagnosed asthma in the pt may make the diagnosis more likely, but be sure
to consider alternative diagnoses if the presentation is not typical.

Has the child been to the ER with this problem before?
Multiple previous ER visits may suggest a more severe or poorly controlled asthma.

Has the child been intubated or in the ICU before?
History of previous intubations or ICU admissions for asthma warrants more
aggressive treatment to prevent reintubation and risk of death.

Does the child have a history of intubation in the NICU?
This suggests possible lung disease such as laryngo- or tracheomalacia or
bronchopulmonary dysplasia. Clinical course can be more severe as a result of less
ability to compensate.

Does the child have frequent nighttime cough?
This may indicate a previously undiagnosed asthma.

**Does anyone else in the family have asthma, eczema, or allergic
rhinitis?**
A family history of allergic disease makes the diagnosis of asthma more likely.

O **Check a pulse oximetry reading and perform a quick, focused PE.**
Quickly assess the pt's level of respiratory distress:

- Unable to speak in full sentences		- Accessory respiratory
- Tachypnea	- Tachycardia	muscle usage
- Low O_2 saturation	- Nasal flaring	- Tripod posture
- Subcostal retractions	- Abdominal breathing	- Suprasternal retractions

To see most of these symptoms, you must expose the pt's chest wall. A common
mistake is the failure to do exactly this. The pt may look very comfortable until you
take the shirt off and see retractions and abdominal breathing.

Listen carefully to the lungs.
Pts with reactive airway disease will typically have:
- *Wheezing:* A high-pitched sound on expiration; indicates lower airway
  obstruction.
- *Poor air movement* (a worrisome sign): Lack of sound with visible chest wall
  excursion.

After treatments, the lungs may actually sound worse, with more wheezing, crackles,
and rhonchi because more of the airways have opened up and are subsequently
making noise.

Obtain a chest x-ray (CXR).

- Hyperinflated lung fields	- Flattened diaphragms	- Lack of infiltrates
- Atelectasis	- Peribronchial cuffing	
- Lobar infiltrates or unilateral pathology suggest other illnesses.		

**If pts can cooperate, have them blow as hard as they can into a peak
flow meter.**
Peak flow will help assess the severity of an acute asthma exacerbation.

A **Asthma (a.k.a. Reactive Airway Disease), acute exacerbation**
Asthma is the most common chronic inflammatory disease of the airways. It is a complex pathologic state in which chronic airway inflammation leads to increased mucus production and bronchoconstriction. Bronchoconstriction causes lower airway obstruction, which is intermittent and reversible with bronchodilators.

Differential diagnosis
Foreign body in the airway if not easily seen on CXR may appear as unilateral hyperinflation of a lung caused by air trapping. The right lung is the more common because the left mainstem bronchus takes off at more of an angle than the right.
Respiratory syncytial virus/viral bronchiolitis: Usually presents with fever and is unlikely to improve with breathing treatments.
Laryngotracheomalacia or bronchopulmonary dysplasia are usually accompanied by a history of a prolonged NICU course with intubation.
Vascular rings and slings are congenital malformations of the aortic arch, which constrict the airway and may lead to wheezing or stridor.

Assess severity of an exacerbation.
If the peak flow is less than 30% of the predicted value, this indicates a severe attack. More than 60% is considered a mild attack. Treat severe attacks more aggressively.

P **Provide supplemental oxygen.**
Until the pt is no longer hypoxic. Maintain oxygen saturation >94%.

Give a short-acting β_2 agonist, such as albuterol.
Begin with a handheld nebulized β_2 agonist (2.5 mg in infants/toddlers, 5 mg in older children/adolescents) in addition to the supplemental oxygen. If the pt improves significantly, repeat as needed. If not, continue with the treatment until improvement occurs.

Give corticosteroids.
Equivalent of 2 mg/kg prednisone per day for 5 days should reduce the inflammation. If you are only treating for 5 days, there is no need to taper the dose.

Admit for:
Only mild improvement with ongoing respiratory distress or hypoxia. The pt will need albuterol q4h with a respiratory check every 2 hrs. If the pt needs continuous albuterol, assess carefully whether pt should be on the regular ward versus in a more monitored setting.
If pt fails to respond or worsens, prepare to transfer to the PICU and consider intubation.

Discharge if:
The pt responds well to treatment with complete resolution of hypoxia, retractions, and other signs of respiratory distress. Prescribe a five-day course of corticosteroids with β_2 agonist as needed. Give clear instructions to the pt's caregivers to return to the ER if symptoms return or if relief medicine (β_2 agonist) is being used regularly without improvement.

Try to assess whether this is intermittent or persistent asthma
If you assess the pt as persistent, be sure to prescribe a controller medication such as an inhaled corticosteroid for daily use. Give clear instructions to the pt (if old enough) and pt's caregivers on proper use of the spacer and inhaler and be sure to provide a clear asthma action plan (see Chronic Cough/Wheeze p. 44).

S **Begin by calming the parent(s) and asking them to describe what happened.**

Parents may run into the ER with a well-appearing baby in a panic because their baby stopped breathing at home.

Typical stories depict an infant whom the parent observes to be suddenly not breathing, grunting, or straining. There will often be a history of facial (especially perioral) color change to pale or blue.

How long did the event last?
It is important to discern for how long the baby seemed not to be breathing.

How did recovery occur?
One should find out if an attempt was made at CPR, or if other attempts at stimulation were made (shaking or backslapping), or if the infant simply recovered spontaneously.

Has anything like this ever occurred before or since?
To get a general idea of whether this baby has a chronic condition, you would want to know a history of similar events. Recent recurrence, on the other hand, would give an indication of an acute process the child is currently undergoing.

Is the baby premature?
Premature infants have underdeveloped respiratory drive centers and poorly developed lungs. Apneas are more common.

Was the child crying forcefully immediately before the episode?
If so, consider a breath-holding spell, a benign syncope in infants and toddlers in which children get so worked up that they literally stop breathing. Loss of consciousness can result. It can be followed by jerking movements and circumoral pallor or cyanosis but always resolves spontaneously.

O **Place the infant on a monitor to check the vitals and oxygen saturation levels.**

Oxygen saturation should be 100%. The infant should be afebrile, heart rate in the 120s to 160s with a respiratory rate in the 30s to 40s.

Check the growth parameters.
Weight or length less than the 5th percentile might indicate failure to thrive.

Head circumference less than the 5th percentile indicates microcephaly. These infants may have underdeveloped brains, which may lead to apneas.

Large infants (greater than 95th percentile) may have been born to diabetic mothers. They are typically immature for their size and may have apneas.

Is there any evidence that the infant is in distress?

- Accessory respiratory muscle usage	- Tachypnea	- Tachycardia
	- Nasal flaring	- Suprasternal retractions
- Low O_2 saturation	- Grunting	- Gasping
- Subcostal retractions		

Perform a full PE, starting with the heart and lungs, proceeding to check capillary refill time and complete the rest of the regular exam.
Lungs: Should sound clear without wheezes, rhonchi, or rales.

Heart: There should be no heart murmurs.

Capillary refill: Should be 1 to 2 seconds.

Facial features: Dysmorphism may indicate a syndromic child.

Anterior fontanelle: Should be flat and soft.
Nares: Should be patent with no mucosal congestion.

Labs
Check CBC and blood cultures to rule out sepsis or other infections.
If in the winter, consider a nasopharyngeal swab to test for respiratory syncytial virus.

A **Apparent Life-Threatening Event, a.k.a. ALTE (pronounced "ahl-tee")**
Any perception by the parent that their child almost died or stopped breathing
is an ALTE.
Only about 2% of children who have ALTEs later go on to have sudden infant death
syndrome. The risk is increased to about 10% if the episode occurred while the child
was sleeping and required a resuscitative effort such as CPR.
Because there is no test to prove that it was a simple benign choking episode caused by
a momentary lapse in swallow coordination, the only way to be safe is to rule out
more dangerous causes such as seizure, decreased respiratory drive caused by a central
nervous system (CNS) abnormality, aspiration, etc.

Differential diagnosis of etiologies of an ALTE:
Infections (25%): RSV, sepsis, meningitis
Gastroesophageal reflux (20%): Causes laryngeal chemoreceptor stimulation
Neurologic disorders (20%): Seizures; CNS anomalies; breath-holding spells
Idiopathic (35%)

P **Admit most ALTEs for workup and monitoring.**
A thorough H&P, CXR, and eventually an EEG and MRI are all warranted.
It is not enough to rule in GERD and say that that was the cause. The dangerous causes
such as seizures, sepsis, and CNS abnormalities need to be ruled out.

**If the history is highly suggestive of a breath-holding spell, this would
be a case where admission and workup are not necessary. Educate the
parent.**
Instruct the parent that the next time the child seems to be crying hard enough to lose
consciousness, to quickly blow air in the child's face. This usually averts an episode.

S **Ask the child, "Where does it hurt most?"**
Have the child point with one finger to the place where it hurts most.

Does the pain radiate, travel, go anywhere else?
Radiation to the jaw or left arm is more consistent with myocardial ischemia (angina).
Radiation to the back is more consistent with pancreatitis or dissecting aorta.
It is unlikely that the child will have any of these problems.

Obtain a good description of the timing of the pain: onset, duration, and frequency.
Cardiac chest pain tends to be of sudden onset, last minutes, and recurs with exertion.
Noncardiac pain lasts only seconds or is chronic, with gradual onset and variable
 recurrence.

What number would you use to describe the pain on a scale of 0 to 10?
Pain scores give an idea of the severity of the pain from the pt's perspective. Keep this
 in mind if the child appears comfortable, without tachycardia, and says the pain is a
 10 out of 10.

How would you describe the pain (sharp, dull, burning, etc.)?
Cardiac pain is usually dull, pressure-like. Sharp, stabbing, or burning pain is less
 worrisome.

Ask what makes the pain worse or better.
Angina: Pain that is worse with eating or exertion
Pericarditis: Pain that is worse with lying down and improved with leaning forward
Musculoskeletal: Pain with chest wall palpation and not associated with exertion
Pain that wakes a child up from sleep is always a worrisome sign

Are any other symptoms associated with the pain?
Possible cardiac symptoms (all can occur with anxiety as well): Sweating, nausea,
 paresthesias in the left arm, palpitations, dizziness, syncope, dyspnea
Respiratory symptoms: Dyspnea, cough, wheeze

Ask if the child has ever had this pain before.
It is always useful to know if this has ever happened in the past, and if so, what became
 of it.

Ask a pertinent past medical history. Red flags include:
- Malignancy	- Rheumatic fever
- Cardiac disease or surgery	- Kawasaki disease

Has anyone in the family had a history of heart problems? Red flags include:
- Cardiomyopathy   - Sudden death in <50-yr-old   - Syncope

O **Perform a physical exam, specifically including:**
Look for any features suggestive of genetic syndromes associated with a cardiac
 anomaly.
Look for vital signs consistent with pain (tachycardia or isolated systolic hypertension).
Palpate and auscultate the chest wall for tenderness, thrill, displaced point of maximal
 impulse, or murmur.

Obtain an ECG.
This will rule out any major cardiac causes and make the pt and parent feel better.

Check other studies to rule out pathology if indicated by the H&P.
Chest x-ray to look at lung fields, heart size, and great arteries

Echocardiogram to check origin of coronary arteries, heart and aortic size, and
   ventricular function
Exercise stress test to look for arrhythmia or ischemia

 Chest pain
Pain can occur for a variety of different reasons, but because myocardial infarction
   (MI) is the number-one killer of adults in the United States, we are often overly
   concerned about this rare possibility in pediatrics. Having said this, keep in mind that
   in rare situations, such as anomalous coronary artery or ectasias caused by Kawasaki
   disease, pediatric MIs are still possible.

Differential diagnosis
Benign adolescent chest pain: 8 to 16 yrs old, symptoms for months, sharp knife-like
   pain, variable severity, occurs at rest, brief paroxysmal episodes, normal PE and ECG
Chest wall (35%): Trauma, herpes zoster, costochondritis, slipping rib, muscle strain
Pulmonary (10%): Asthma, pneumothorax, pulmonary embolus, pneumonia
GI (5%): GERD, odynophagia, esophageal spasm, pancreatitis, biliary colic
Psychogenic (10–30%): Hyperventilation syndrome, anxiety attack, stress
Unknown (10%)

Check the ECG for ST segment elevations corresponding to different coronary arteries (Table 5):
If you see ST segment elevations in any of the above patterns, strongly consider MI. If
   the ST segment elevation is in all leads, consider pericarditis.
Evaluate the ECG for ventricular hypertrophy, long QT (>0.45 sec), or arrhythmia.
A normal ECG does not rule out a cardiac etiology, but it does make it less likely.

Table 5 ECG Results

I	H	aVR	X	V1	S	V4	A
II	I	aVL	H	V2	S	V5	L
III	I	aVF	I	V3	A	V6	L

High Lateral corresponds to I & aVL   =   Left Circumflex
Inferior corresponds to II, III, & aVF =   Right Coronary Artery
Septal corresponds to V1 & V2   =   Left Anterior Descending Septal Branch
Anterior corresponds to V3 & V4   =   LAD Diagonal Branch
Lateral corresponds to V5 & V6   =   Left Circumflex

P **If you suspect noncardiac pain, perform tests to diagnose and treat causes appropriately. If the pain is psychogenic, give reassurance and refer to psychiatry.**
More than 95% of chest pain pts will be like this. Reassure and send them home.

If the pain is cardiac, monitor the pt carefully and consult Cardiology for intervention.

If you suspect MI, give supplemental O$_2$, sublingual nitroglycerine, aspirin, and if necessary, morphine to control the pain. Check a serum troponin level.
A good mnemonic to remember this is **MONA**.
Troponin is a cardiac enzyme. It is present if there is myocardial injury.

S **When did the symptoms start, and where is the pain located?**
If the pain is long-standing, consider constipation, irritable bowel syndrome (IBS), or possibly inflammatory bowel disease (IBD). For more acute processes, the location is very important:
Generalized: Small bowel obstruction (SBO), Henoch-Schönlein purpura, constipation, IBS, IBD, colitis, gas
RUQ: Hepatitis, cholecystitis, choledocholithiasis, liver abscess
LUQ: Peptic ulcer disease, gastritis, pancreatitis
Periumbilical: Pancreatitis, appendicitis, Meckel's diverticulum
Flank: Pyelonephritis, kidney stone
RLQ: Appendicitis, Meckel's diverticulum, colitis/IBD
LLQ: Meckel's diverticulum, constipation, colitis/IBD
Suprapubic: Urinary tract infection (UTI)
Pelvic: In adolescent females, is associated with a wide differential, including:
- Pelvic inflammatory disease (PID)   - Ovarian torsion
- Endometriosis   - Mittelschmerz

What are the associated symptoms?
Fever, vomiting, and/or diarrhea: Appendicitis, cholecystitis, Henoch-Schönlein purpura, pyelonephritis, hepatitis, liver abscess, UTI, PID
Bilious (dark green) emesis: SBO or ileus
Bloody emesis: Peptic ulcer disease
Bloody stool: Colitis/IBD, Meckel's diverticulum, intussusception

When was the pt's last normal bowel movement (BM)?
Important for generating the differential diagnosis. No BMs versus diarrhea suggests different entities.

O **How old is the pt and is he or she the appropriate size?**
Age is also an important factor in making diagnoses such as pyloric stenosis more or less likely.
Pts with chronic inflammatory processes are usually small for age.

Perform a PE.
Some illnesses that can mimic abdominal complaints include:
- *Group A strep pharyngitis:* Causes a mesenteric adenitis, mimicking an appendicitis
- *Pneumonia:* Can cause RUQ or LUQ pain
- *Testicular torsions:* Radiate to the lower quadrants

Does the pt have a surgical or nonsurgical abdomen?
Surgical abdomens (suggesting diseases that will require surgery) imply peritonitis:
- *Guarding:* The abdominal musculature will contract on palpation of the area with pain.
- *Rebound:* Pain occurring when you abruptly remove your fingers after palpating deeply.
- *Percussion tenderness:* Significant pain with tapping abdominal wall.
- *Pain with movement:* Pts with peritoneal inflammation hold very still. If the pt is writhing in pain, it is less likely to be a surgical abdomen. If you are uncertain, have the pt jump up and down (if it is a child) or have the mother bounce the pt on her knee (if it is a toddler). If this is tolerated without pain, surgical abdomen is unlikely.

Although the entire abdomen may be tender, there is usually a point of maximal tenderness:
- *RLQ:* Appendicitis
- *Epigastrium:* Perforated peptic ulcer disease
- *RUQ:* Cholecystitis
- *Periumbilical area:* SBO, pancreatitis (pancreatitis will rarely require surgery)

Perform specific tests for appendicitis, if it is suspected.
Rovsing's sign: Palpation anywhere in the abdomen causes pain in the RLQ.
Psoas sign: Hyperextending the right leg at the hip causes pain.
Obturator sign: With the right leg flexed at the knee and hip, abducting the hip worsens pain.
Rectal: Palpation of the right rectal wall is exquisitely tender.

Perform an abdominal x-ray (Kidney-Ureter-Bladder or KUB).
This will not always give you the diagnosis, but it may show an RLQ fecalith in the case of appendicitis, calcifications in the case of kidney stones, or distended loops of bowel in an SBO.

A ### Rule Out Appendicitis.
Appendicitis can occur at any age but is most common near adolescence.
Most common cause of abdominal pain requiring surgery in children.
Results from an obstructed, infected appendix with pus and pressure.
Presentation is variable, but it commonly begins with periumbilical pain and then vomiting and loss of appetite. In several hours, the pain moves to the RLQ and the pt will hold still so as to not exacerbate the pain. If left untreated, the pain worsens, comes to a climax, and then improves as the appendix perforates. If still left untreated, pain will again worsen and the pt may become septic. If an abscess cannot be walled off, death may follow.

Differential diagnosis
As can be implied from the subjective portion of this SOAP, the differential diagnosis is massive. If the pt has an H&P consistent with appendicitis, consider:
- Constipation
- Colitis
- Mittelschmerz
- PID
- Ovarian torsion

P **If the abdomen is surgical, call the surgery team immediately to evaluate it. These pts should be admitted. If the abdomen is nonsurgical, further diagnostic tests include:**
Blood for CBC, chemistry panel (Na, K, Cl, HCO_3, BUN, Cr, Glucose; especially if the pt has been vomiting), liver panel, amylase, and lipase (elevated in the case of pancreatitis)
- Elevated WBC count, neutrophilia, or bandemia on CBC are all consistent with an inflammatory process but are very nonspecific.

Check a U/A.
Leukocyte esterase and nitrites positive suggest a UTI.
Blood could indicate a stone or Henoch-Schönlein purpura.

Perform an U/S and/or CT of the abdomen and pelvis if still unsure of the diagnosis.
Appendicitis is sometimes seen. Other diagnoses may also be made this way.

S **How old is the child? How long has this been going on?**

Pyloric stenosis usually occurs at about 2 to 4 weeks of age but may be seen up to 3 months old.

Emesis will usually start around the second to third week of life and progressively worsen.

How long after feeding does the child vomit? How many times per day?

Vomiting should occur within about half an hour of every, or nearly every, feed.

Is the vomiting truly projectile?

The vomiting should be described as traveling some distance, possibly across the room.

What is the color of the emesis?

Emesis should look like the recently consumed milk. It should not be dark yellow or green. This would imply the presence of bile in the emesis, which would suggest another diagnosis.

Is the pt a boy or a girl, and is there a family history of pyloric stenosis?

For some reason, boys are more likely (4:1) than girls to have pyloric stenosis.

There is also often a parent or close family member with a history of surgery in infancy.

O **Examine the child carefully. Look for the peristaltic wave and the olive.**

Observe the feeding and subsequent vomiting if you are able to. The baby should appear hungry during the feeding but forcefully vomit the feed within about half an hour.

Look at the child's abdomen and watch the epigastrium for the peristaltic wave.

Examine the abdomen for the olive by holding the infant's knees up toward it's chest. Palpate in the epigastrium for a discrete, mobile mass about the size and shape of an olive.

Look for signs of dehydration and assess degree of dehydration.

See Dehydration p. 130. A dehydrated baby is consistent with the diagnosis.

Check an abdominal plain film x-ray.

A gas-filled stomach with little gas elsewhere supports the diagnosis of pyloric stenosis.

Obtain an U/S of the abdomen.

U/S is the best modality with which to look for pyloric hypertrophy. The pylorus should be ≥5 mm wide and ≥15 mm long to be consistent with pyloric stenosis.

Check a stat chem 7 and a U/A.

Hypochloremic alkalosis: Frequent emesis causes a loss of electrolytes produced in the stomach, mainly chloride and hydrogen, increasing serum bicarbonate and potassium.

Hypokalemia: In the presence of low intravascular volume, aldosterone increases the renal uptake of sodium and wastes potassium and hydrogen. As a result, serum K^+ is usually low.

Paradoxical aciduria: Despite the apparent metabolic alkalosis (elevated serum bicarbonate), the urine pH will be low. Aldosterone increases H^+ excretion to preserve intravascular volume.

A   Pyloric Stenosis

This phenomenon occurs in infants at the end of their neonatal period in which the pyloric musculature becomes hypertrophied and ingestions cannot pass. It is usually idiopathic, and the natural history is that it would resolve in 1 to 2 months if left alone. Unfortunately, it would be difficult for the infant to survive that long untreated. Surgery is the better option.

Differential Diagnosis

Gastroesophageal reflux: Must differentiate between true vomiting and spitting up.

Metabolic disorder: Poor weight gain and emesis

Malrotation/volvulus: Can happen at any age, but is common in this age group. It is differentiated from pyloric stenosis by its bilious emesis and intermittent symptoms. If it is missed, midgut volvulus can compromise blood flow, causing necrotic bowel. Death follows.

Appendicitis: Rarely diagnosed clinically in pts less than 1 yr old but has an extremely atypical and serious presentation in this age group because of the inability of the child to talk and the lack of a well-developed omentum to localize the infection.

Duodenal atresia/stenosis: Will generally present with bilious emesis in the NICU.

Necrotizing enterocolitis: Mostly premature babies in the NICU with vomiting, feeding intolerance, heme-positive stools, and radiographic findings (see NEC p. 22).

Hernia or adhesions: Any hernia that becomes incarcerated or adhesions after abdominal surgery can cause a small bowel obstruction, which is associated with bilious vomiting resulting from the dilated proximal small bowel.

Enteritis: Causes large, voluminous, watery stools often resulting from viruses (like rotavirus and the noroviruses) and bacteria (like *E. coli* (not O157 H7), *Vibrio cholerae*, and salmonella). The vomiting is caused by distention of the small bowel with the voluminous diarrhea. There may be an associated fever (see Vomiting and Diarrhea p. 76).

UTI: Many infants with urinary tract infections will vomit, likely secondary to the ileus caused by bowel touching the inflamed bladder or kidney. Fever should be present.

Meningitis: Central vomiting can occur with meningitis caused by any infectious agent but is especially prevalent in viral meningitis. Again, one should see fever.

P   Admit this pt. Assess the degree of dehydration and correct it intravenously.

See Dehydration and Intravenous Fluid Management p. 130. Maintenance fluids can be started when the dehydration improves.

Make the child NPO, place a nasogastric tube to gravity, and consult a surgeon.

After a variable time, decompressing the stomach and getting it to relax some from all of its recent activity, the surgeons will perform a pylorotomy.

- *Pylorotomy:* Involves cutting along the pylorus transversely and sewing it up horizontally, relieving some of the stenosis. The surgery is usually curative, and the child will slowly begin to eat over the next few days and then completely recover with usually no residual sequelae.

See Postop Care of the Pyloric Stenosis Patient p. 136.

S **How long has the child been vomiting? Having diarrhea? How many times per day?**

When the pt presents with what may be enteritis, it is important to differentiate it from other possible causes of vomiting and diarrhea.

The time course is important; it is almost always vomiting before diarrhea. Consider alternative diagnoses if:

- *Vomiting follows diarrhea:* Colitis with sepsis, hemolytic uremic syndrome (HUS)
- *Diarrhea never appears:* Pyelonephritis, meningitis, appendicitis

The number of times of each episode per day indicates the severity of the disease.

Is the child's urine output decreased?

A decrease in the average number of wet diapers or voids suggests dehydration.

What is the color of the emesis/diarrhea? Is there blood or bile present in the emesis or blood present in the stool?

Bloody emesis: Suggests an upper gastrointestinal bleed. This may be a component of enteritis, but it can also suggest something more serious.

Bilious emesis: Suggests an intestinal obstruction, often associated with decreased stooling, not diarrhea.

Diarrhea can be many different colors, but frank blood suggests a lower GI bleed, possibly colitis (see Bloody Diarrhea p. 78). Mucus in the stool also suggests colitis.

Black stool: Suggests an occult upper GI bleed.

Is the child keeping any oral intake down?

This is the most important question; if all of the other questions are missed, this must be asked. All therapy is based on hydrating the child.

O **What are the vital signs?**

Tachycardia indicates a volume-depleted infant. Children can have a normal BP until shortly before cardiovascular collapse. Fever may be present but is less common than with colitis.

How does the child look?

General appearance: A happy, playful child, or a child actively resisting the doctor is likely to be better hydrated than a weak-appearing child with poor coloring.

Hydration: Palpate the fontanelle (if less than 1 yr old), assess tear production, assess lips and buccal mucosa for moisture, and capillary refill time.

- Anterior fontanelles may be sunken with dehydration.
- Dehydrated children do not produce tears. This sign is unreliable in infants younger than 3 months.
- The lips and oral mucosa should appear moist and not tacky.
- Push down over the child's heel or great toe and release. Count the number of seconds until the pink color returns. Less than 2 seconds is normal.

Send the blood for electrolytes and BUN and creatinine.

If the pt has been vomiting and having a lot of diarrhea, he or she could easily have electrolyte abnormalities or acute renal failure.

Send the stool for viral and bacterial culture.

Rotavirus can be tested for using an enzyme-linked immunoassay of the stool.

The only reasons to send stool for ova and parasites are if the pt is immunocompromised or if you suspect *Giardia* or *Entamoeba*.

Enteritis

If the pt has large, voluminous, watery diarrhea, it is likely to be enteritis. The next step is to consider what organism is causing it:

Viral: (viruses are usually the cause of enteritis)

- *Rotavirus:* Increased incidence in winter and in children 6 months to 3 yrs old. Vomiting usually precedes diarrhea, and there may be mild AST/ALT elevation.
- *Norovirus:* Used to be classified as Norwalk viruses, but this is a whole family of viruses that cause enteritis. This form of enteritis is not seasonal and has the same attack rate in all ages. Often associated with outbreaks at gatherings such as picnics or on cruise ships.
- *Adenovirus:* Although they are more rare, adenoviruses can cause enteritis, but they are more commonly associated with upper respiratory tract infections.

Bacteria:

- *Salmonella:* Need more than 5,000 organisms to cause infection. Often associated with raw eggs, ice cream, and people with pet turtles or salamanders. The diarrhea can be bloody.
- *E. coli:* Not $O_{157}H_7$ (causes colitis and HUS) but rather ETEC (Enterotoxogenic *E. coli*).
- *Vibrio cholerae:* Massive, up to 10 liters per day! Nonexistent outside of the third world.

Protozoa: Giardia actually causes a duodenitis, which leads to large, smelly, fatty stools with bloating, cramping, and gas. It would rarely be confused with enteritis.

Differential diagnosis

       - Colitis   - Appendicitis   - UTI   - HUS   - Meningitis

Assess degree of dehydration.

See Dehydration and Intravenous Fluid Management p. 130.

If the child tolerates oral liquid at home and the PE reveals a well-hydrated or 5% dehydrated child, reassure the parents.

The child will do well as long as he or she continues to take liquids. Solids will return in time.

If the parents state that the child keeps no oral liquid down, begin oral liquids 1 teaspoon at a time.

If the child takes oral liquid in the ER, he or she may be sent home with instructions on slow hydration.

For 10% to 15% dehydration, or if the pt fails the oral liquid trial (emesis within 30 minutes), start 20 cc/kg normal saline IV bolus. Draw stat electrolytes while the IV is being placed.

Continue IV normal saline until the child makes urine and the appearance improves.

For 15% dehydration and a lethargic child, obtain emergent venous access via an intraosseous line (tibia) bolus NS as above.

A child in this state is on the verge of cardiovascular collapse.

Admit for:

Failure to tolerate oral liquid, >5% dehydration, or continuing to appear ill after receiving IV fluids.

S When did the diarrhea start? How many times per day? Large or small amount? Is there any blood or mucus in the stool? Is there any vomiting?

Gastroenteritis, as it is commonly called, is actually a misnomer because there is no stomach inflammation associated with the vomiting. In reality, there are two clinical entities:

- *Enteritis:* Few, voluminous, watery, nonbloody stools without mucus, preceded by vomiting. It is more common and more benign.
- *Colitis:* Small, frequent, bloody stools with mucus, rarely with vomiting.

These questions will help you distinguish the two.

Is there abdominal pain?

Colitis is often associated with crampy belly pain and tenesmus.

Did the child eat anything out of the ordinary recently?

Because food poisoning is a possible cause of this condition, eating food from street vendors, a restaurant, or just something questionably old from the refrigerator are all useful clues.

Has the child traveled anywhere recently?

Travel increases the risk for an exotic parasitic or bacterial infection.

Is anyone else sick at home?

If other people, both children and adults, are also suffering from this same problem, it is another suggestion that this may be infectious diarrhea.

Is the child's urine output normal or decreased?

This question is a quick way to assess the hydration status of the child.

O Perform a PE and review of the vital signs.

Vital signs: Tachycardia indicates a volume-depleted infant. Children can have a normal BP until shortly before cardiovascular collapse. Fever is common.

General appearance: A happy, playful child, or a child actively resisting the doctor is likely to be better hydrated than a weak, pale-appearing child.

Hydration: Palpate the fontanelle (if less than 1 yr old), assess tear production, assess lips and buccal mucosa for moisture, and capillary refill time.

- Anterior fontanelles may be sunken with dehydration.
- Lack of tears suggests dehydration unless the patient is <3 months old.
- The lips and oral mucosa should appear moist and not tacky.
- Push down over the child's heel or great toe and release. Count the number of seconds until the pink color returns. Less than 2 seconds is normal.

Order appropriate lab tests.

Check a CBC. It rarely makes a diagnosis but may help in the following areas:

- WBC count is more likely to be elevated with colitis than enteritis.
- Anemia may suggest prolonged bleeding (iron deficiency) or chronic inflammation.
- Eosinophilia can suggest a parasitic infection.

An erythrocyte sedimentation rate is helpful if autoimmune colitis is suspected.

Check stool for WBCs and occult blood. A guaiac may be performed in the ER to check the latter. Both can be signs of colonic inflammation.

A stool bacterial culture is always a must if colitis is even suspected. If there is still a possibility that this could be enteritis, rotavirus studies may be sent. If the pt is immunocompromised, add a cytomegalovirus (CMV) viral culture as well.

If you suspect parasitic infection, check the stool for ova and parasites (O&P).
Check the stool for *Clostridium difficile* toxin if the patient has been on antibiotics.

A Colitis

Bacterial causes:

- *Shigella:* Only infects humans, does not enter bloodstream (septicemia), and is associated with seizures caused by shigatoxin. WBC is mildly elevated with significant left shift (bandemia). Treat with ceftriaxone or Bactrim to reduce the carrier-state.
- *Salmonella:* Can infect animals such as chickens and turtles and can enter the bloodstream and cause septicemia, especially *Salmonella typhae*. If enteric or typhoid fever is present, it may be without diarrhea with a low (<4000) WBC. Antibiotics may increase the carrier-state.
- *Campylobacter:* Number-one cause of colitis. It is associated with Guillain-Barré syndrome. Treat with macrolide antibiotics.
- *E. coli* $O_{157}H_7$: Associated with hemolytic uremic syndrome (HUS), which is intravascular hemolysis (schistocytes on peripheral smear), acute renal failure, and thrombocytopenia. Do not give antibiotics because this increases the chances and severity of HUS.
- *Yersinia enterocolitica:* Presentation can mimic appendicitis.
- *Clostridium difficile:* Antibiotics kill the usually protective commensurate organisms in the bowel. The clostridia then grow and secrete a toxin that creates a pseudomembrane over the normal mucosa. Hence the name pseudomembranous colitis.

Parasitic causes:

- *Entamoeba histolytica:* The only reason to check O&P if your host is immunocompetent.
- Infectious worms can cause disease, but unless your patient has traveled to an endemic area, these should be thought of as rare causes.

Immunosuppressed patient: Think of cryptosporidia, microsporidia, isospora, cryptococcus, mycobacterium-avium complex, and CMV.

Inflammatory bowel disease (IBD) such as Crohn's disease or ulcerative colitis is the main noninfectious cause of colitis.

Differential diagnosis

- Appendicitis	- Meckel's diverticulum	- Intussusception
- Milk protein allergy	- Enteritis	

P Treat hypovolemia/dehydration if present.

See Dehydration and Intravenous Fluid Management p. 130.

For shigella and campylobacter, give antibiotics but exclude *E. coli* $O_{157}H_7$ and salmonella.

Treat pseudomembranous colitis and *Entamoeba histolytica* with oral metronidazole.

Call a gastroenterology specialist for suspected IBD.

Admit the child if:

He or she is dehydrated and not taking oral liquids, if there are signs of sepsis (tachycardia and hypotension not responsive to IV fluids), or if this is a chronic problem.

Consider admission to the PICU for suspected HUS.

S

What symptoms was the child having at home?

Intussusception (a condition in which one portion of the bowel moves into one
another, a.k.a. telescoping) initially presents as paroxysms of abdominal pain, with an
infant screaming or crying. During these paroxysms, the infant will often appear to be
straining, drawing the knees up to the abdomen.

Between paroxysms, the infant may appear to be well, playing and acting normally.
Later the pt is lethargic and occasionally even encephalopathic between paroxysms.
Emesis, especially bilious emesis, is very common.

The parent may also note bloody stools. These stools are often bright red blood mixed
with mucus and are called currant-jelly stools because of their resemblance to dark
reddish jelly.

How old is the pt?

It is more common in infants but can occur at any age and is extremely uncommon in
neonates; 60% of all cases occur in the first year of life, usually between 4 and
10 months; 80% of all cases occur before the second birthday.

Has the child been recently ill with any other conditions?

It is often associated with a recent infection (especially adenovirus):

     - Otitis media   - Gastroenteritis   - Upper respiratory infection

Noninfectious predisposing events include:

     - Henoch-Schönlein purpura   - Bezoar   - Lymphoma

All of these conditions can cause enlargement of the terminal ileal lymph clusters
known as Peyer's patches, forming a lead point that is caught up in the peristaltic
wave of the intestine and causes a proximal piece to be moved distally, often through
the ileocecal valve.

O

Check the vital signs.

Tachycardia and tachypnea, secondary to pain. Fever can be very high, up to 106°F.

As noted above, these pts might have unstable vitals. If the tachycardia and tachypnea
are associated with dropping blood pressures, call for help immediately.

Perform a PE, paying particular attention to the abdomen.

A careful exam of the abdomen may reveal a tender sausage-shaped mass, usually in the
RUQ. It may increase in size during a paroxysm of pain.

Intussusception usually begins at the ileocecal valve.

- Dance's sign is an empty RLQ on exam caused by intussusception of enough
  bowel to reach the transverse colon.

Perform a rectal exam.

If the entire colon is intussuscepted, the advancing intestine may prolapse through the
anus.

Look on the finger of your glove for bloody mucus (current-jelly stool). This is highly
suggestive, but its absence does not exclude intussusception.

Perform an abdominal x-ray series.

There may be dilated loops of small bowel or a paucity of bowel gas. There may even be
a soft tissue mass in the area of the intussusception.

Check a CBC.

A WBC count between 10,000 and 18,000 is common.

If you are still not convinced, obtain an abdominal U/S.
A tubular mass can be seen in longitudinal view and a doughnut-shaped mass in transverse view.

A Intussusception

Intussusception is a common condition, but it can be lethal if misdiagnosed. When the bowel telescopes, it drags its mesentery with it, which becomes constricted in the tight loop of bowel. This leads to poor venous return, further swelling, and more constriction. The currant-jelly stool is caused by leaking of blood from this engorged bowel. If this process is allowed to continue, the bowel will eventually die and become necrotic from lack of blood supply and the oxygen it carries. Necrotic bowel must be removed or the pt will die.

Differential diagnosis

- Malrotation   - Volvulus   - Appendicitis
- Enteritis   - Colitis   - Obstruction
- Mesenteric adenitis   - Mesenteric ischemia   - Biliary tract stenosis
- Renal stones   - Ileus
- Acidosis (as in diabetic ketoacidosis)
- Gastroesophageal reflux disorder
- Pelvic inflammatory disease

- Bowel obstruction has a subdifferential including:
  - Stool   - Bezoar   - Parasites
  - Stricture   - Tumor/lymphatic tissue

Intussusception can also be mistaken for meningitis because of the lethargy occurring between paroxysms and the associated high fever.

In pts who are out of the usual age range, or who are having a recurrent intussusception, evaluate for a possible pathologic lead point.
Lead points include:

- Inverted appendiceal stump   - Meckel's diverticulum   - Intestinal polyp
- Duplication   - Lymphoma   - Sarcoma

Rarely, intussusception will be the first sign of cystic fibrosis because it can happen to these pts when they become dehydrated.

P Send the pt for an emergent barium or air-contrast enema.

Before U/S, barium enema was the diagnostic procedure of choice. It shows barium leaking around the intussuscepted bowel in a coil-spring appearance; however, it was also noted that the hydrostatic pressure built up behind the telescoping bowel often reduced the intussusception.

If performed within the first 48 hrs, reduction occurs in approximately 75% to 80% of pts. After 48 hrs, this number drops to 50%.

Air contrast has reduced the rates of perforation from 0.5% to 2.5% with barium to <0.2%.

If the enema does not work, call an emergent surgery consult.
The pt will require an emergent laparotomy to attempt surgical reduction. If reduction seems impossible during surgery, or if the bowel already seems necrotic, the intussusception will be excised and an end-to-end anastomosis performed.

Ileo-ileal intussusception (rare) is unlikely to reduce with enema, and most require surgery.

S **Ask the parents if they know what their child took.**

All of the following differ in threat to life and type of supportive care required. Some of these toxins even have an antidote:

- Medications   - Cleaning agents   - Alcohol
- Hydrocarbons (like gasoline)   - Illicit drugs   - Lead paint   - Plants

If the parents identify the toxin as a medication, but do not know what type, or state that multiple open pill bottles were found, ask what kinds of meds are in the house or what kinds of medical conditions the people who live in the house have.

This line of questioning will help narrow down the field of possible drugs.
If possible, have someone bring in the pills and bottles that are left.

When did the ingestion occur?

Many actions you may take depend on how long it has been since the ingestion.

If the pt is an adolescent, it is important to ask if the ingestion was intentional.

Perform a HEADSS exam with the parent(s) out of the room (see WCC: Adolescent p. 40).

Has the child had any symptoms?

- Change in mental status   - Vomiting   - Fevers
- Seizures   - Headaches

O **Evaluate the pt's general appearance.**

Often the pt will either appear well (most common) or altered/obtunded. Emergently evaluate the obtunded pt, and if the gag reflex is not present or the Glasgow Coma Score <8, intubate.

Perform a rapid, but general PE. Attempt to identify certain "toxidromes," recognizable clusters of symptoms and signs that occur with certain poisonings.

Anticholinergics and sympathomimetics: Pupillary dilation (mydriasis), tachycardia, low-grade fever, urinary retention

- *Anticholinergics* (belladonna, atropine, Jimson weed): Flushing, dry mucous membranes, altered mental status, decreased bowel sounds
- *Sympathomimetics* (cocaine, methamphetamine): Diaphoresis, increased bowel sounds

Cholinergics (insecticides, succinylcholine, pilocarpine) opposite of anticholinergics: Diaphoresis, pupillary contraction (miosis), wheezing, bradycardia, diarrhea, hyperactive bowel sounds, urinary incontinence, excess pulmonary secretions

Salicylates: Tinnitus, nausea, anion gap acidosis, vomiting, tachypnea (to the point of respiratory alkalosis), ketonuria

Opiates (morphine, fentanyl): Nystagmus, miosis, decreased mental status, bradypnea

Tricyclic antidepressants (amitriptyline, nortriptyline, imipramine): Seizures, acidosis, coma, hypotension, tachyarrhythmias, prolonged QRS complex

Phenothiazines (haloperidol, chlorpromazine): Dystonia, fever, rigidity, tremor, oculogyric crisis, prolonged QT, coma

Caustic ingestion (lye, acid, cleaners): Check mouth/lips for evidence of burns.

Check labs.

Check serum and urine toxicology screens (include acetaminophen and aspirin levels if unknown ingestion) and also check liver and renal function.
Check chem 7 for acidosis. Calculate anion gap = $Na - (Cl + HCO_3)$. Normal is <15.

Check an ABG to assess acid–base balance. A low bicarb, with a high pCO_2, may suggest compensation. High pCO_2 or low pO_2 suggests respiratory failure, a need for intubation.

Check an abdominal x-ray.
Rarely, pill fragments are visible. These include:

- Calcium   - Iodine   - Enteric-coated tabs
- Iron   - Heavy metals   - Other foreign bodies

Check an ECG.
Evaluate for arrhythmias or conduction delays.

A Chemical Ingestion
Approximately 50% to 60% of all poisonings are in children younger than 6 yrs old. Toddlers are most common.
Highest rate of suicide attempts is in adolescents. Many attempt poisoning.

Differential diagnosis
A conscious pt may report ingestion and look otherwise well, in which case you investigate the type of ingestion and attempt to limit possible toxicity.

For a comatose pt in whom you have suspected or reported ingestion, be sure to consider other causes of acute coma, such as: (mnemonic VEGO TIPS MD)
- Hypo*V*olemia   - *T*amponade/Hypo*T*hermia   -*M*I
- *E*lectrolyte abnormalities - *I*nternal Bleed (head, abdomen, leg) -*D*rugs
- Hypo*G*lycemia   - *P*neumothorax/Pulmonary
- Hyp*O*xia   embolism
                            - *S*eizure

P Call your local Poison Control Center.

Give activated charcoal 1–2 g/kg to bind organic toxins.
Ineffective against alcohols and things that do not contain carbon, such as caustics, arsenic, bromide, potassium, ethanol, methanol, ethylene glycol, heavy metals, iron, iodine, and lithium.
Syrup of Ipecac is no longer recommended. Have activated charcoal at home instead.
Gastric lavage ("pumping the stomach") is not commonly used anymore but may be used up to 1 hr after ingestion. Do not use with hydrocarbons or caustics.

Antidotes
- Acetaminophen: N-Acetylcysteine
- Benzodiazepine: Flumazenil
- Coumadin: Fresh frozen plasma, vitamin K
- Digitalis: Specific Fab antibody fragments
- Heparin: Protamine sulfate
- Isoniazid: Pyridoxine
- Methemoglobinemia: Methylene blue
- Organophosphates: Atropine/pralidoxime

- Arsenic, lead: Penicillamine
- Carbon monoxide: Oxygen (Hyperbaric)
- Cyanide: Sodium nitrite
- Ethylene glycol/methanol: Ethanol
- Iron: Deferoxamine
- Mercury: BAL
- Narcotics: Naloxone
- Phenothiazines: Diphenhydramine

All suicidal pts must be admitted for psychiatric hold.
See WCC: Adolescent p. 40.

S **What was the foreign body and when and where was it placed?**

Children place foreign bodies (FBs) in just about any orifice.

Usually the nose in <3 yrs old.

Usually the ear in 3 to 8 yrs old.

Starting from the top: Ears, nose, mouth (trachea or esophagus), urethra, vagina, anus, other (trach, g-tube)

O **Do the appropriate general and then focused physical exams and imaging.**

The younger the child, and especially in infants, sometimes there is a history of an FB, but often there will just be symptoms of respiratory distress, drooling, crying with pain, or vaginal discharge, etc. In these cases, it is wise to keep foreign body on your differential.

Esophageal (Round on AP, Flat on Lat): The FB on chest or lateral neck x-ray is seen in the coronal plane. Usually accompanied by dysphagia, drooling, or substernal chest pain.

Tracheal/Bronchial (Tracheal or Laryngeal FBs are seen in the sagittal plane: Flat on AP, Round on Lat): Presents as cough, stridor, hemoptysis, aphonia, or respiratory distress. Decreased breath sounds or wheeze on one side suggests bronchial foreign body (usually the right mainstem bronchus because it branches at less of an angle than the left). Auscultate and percuss lung fields and then get a chest x-ray and AP and lateral neck x-rays looking for tracheal or bronchial foreign body.

Ear/Nose: Unilateral nose or ear pain or foul-smelling discharge or bleeding. Check nose or ears with otoscope for foreign body.

Vaginal: Vaginal bleeding or foul-smelling discharge. Check vaginal exam and consider KUB or U/S to help confirm the diagnosis.

A **Foreign body ingestion versus placement**

Infants put everything in their mouths, so it is the adult caretaker's responsibility to keep things small enough to choke on away from the baby.

Older children usually will just say they were playing and it happened, but sometimes you will get a response that they were suicidal or another child did it to them.

Consider implications of where and what was found in the child.

Infants:

- Oral foreign body: Consider issues of poor supervision, but recognize that it may happen with even the most careful parent.
- With foreign body anywhere else, such as the ear, nose, vagina, g-tube, or tracheostomy, consider abuse (anyone with access to the child such as a caretaker or an older child), especially in children less than 4 months old because they are not usually capable of placing the foreign body themselves.

Older children:

- For a foreign body placed in the rectum, urethra, or vagina (unless it is toilet paper, which is common), consider sexual abuse by anyone with access to the child.
- With repetitive foreign body placement anywhere, consider depression, abuse, or other psychological problem.

P **Remove foreign body.**

Ear canal: Foreign bodies can be removed with a wire loop, alligator forceps, irrigation (except if suspect tympanic membrane perforation or vegetable matter), or suction.

Be careful not to manipulate too much because inflammation can cause the ear canal to swell and make extraction very difficult. If extraction is not made with the first or second attempt, refer to ENT. If it is a live insect, drown it in mineral oil before extraction.

Nasal: Foreign bodies can be removed by first anesthetizing with lidocaine spray and then decreasing inflammation/swelling with phenylephrine drops. Then, when the swelling is decreased, pass a small Foley catheter beyond the foreign body, inflate the balloon, and pull gently back out of the nose. If this does not work, refer to ENT.

Esophageal: Foreign bodies need to be identified as sharp or dull by x-ray (or history if not radiopaque). If it is sharp, get another chest x-ray/KUB to verify passage to stomach and then again in a week to verify passage. Have pt return if any signs of abdominal pain, vomiting, or distention. If the FB is dull, make sure it is not a battery (these can be toxic). If not, instruct to return only if vomiting or abdominal pain occurs. If it is a battery or sharp object and it is stuck in the esophagus, arrange for endoscopic removal. If the battery or sharp is in the stomach, recheck in 24 hrs to assure that it passes the pylorus, but return sooner if there is increasing abdominal pain or vomiting.

Trachea: Keep in position of comfort until ENT or Pulmonary can remove FB. Prepare to manage airway if pt develops severe airway obstruction.

If you suspect abuse or neglect, refer the child to Protective Services.
Do not feel guilty about referring a possible innocent parent to Social Services; even a suspicion may be enough to save a child's life.

If you suspect depression or a suicide, admit pt for a psychiatric hold and call a child psychiatry consult.
If depression is missed, there is a risk that a teen will succeed at suicide in the future.

If you suspect good parents with bad luck, provide preventive education.

S

Where is the edema?
- Periorbital   - Abdominal   - Lower extremities
- Scrotal   - Vulvar   - Scalp

When did the edema begin?
Usually, the edema is worse in the mornings and has been slowly getting worse each day.

When the child urinates in the toilet, does he or she make bubbles or foam?
If there is protein in the urine (proteinuria), urine will be foamy.

Does anyone in the family have renal disease or kidney problems?
If the pt has a strong family history of renal problems such as renal failure or kidney transplant, it is important to take that into account when evaluating.

Does the pt have any other associated symptoms?
Signs such as fever, rash, arthritis, or arthralgias suggest systemic disease such as:
- Lupus   - Vasculitis
- Juvenile rheumatoid arthritis   - Crohn's disease

O

Perform a good general exam.
Plot carefully on the growth curve and evaluate for possible failure to thrive.
Look carefully at the vital signs for hypertension or other clues of renal disease.
Look also at the temperature and exam for signs of infection.
Look specifically at the areas that become edematous in nephrotic syndrome (NS), such as periorbital, scrotal, sacral, ankles, and earlobes (soft, doughy earlobe suggests NS).

Order the appropriate tests for workup of the three main criteria of nephrotic syndrome:
Proteinuria: Check a spot and/or 24-hr urine for protein to creatinine ratio.
Hypoalbuminemia: Check the blood albumin level.
Edema: On physical exam

Perform a urine dipstick.
The presence of large protein suggests the diagnosis of nephrotic syndrome.
Blood may or may not be positive, but remember that hematuria with mild to moderate proteinuria is more consistent with nephritis than nephrosis.

Draw blood for CBC with differential, BUN/Cr, and a lipid panel.
The CBC will reveal both elevated hematocrit and signs of infection.
NS is associated with hyperlipidemia, often considered a 4th criterion.
BUN/Cr rule out renal insufficiency/failure.

Place a PPD.
So that PPD status can be ascertained before starting steroids.

Check for possible alternative or secondary causes with:
Antinuclear antibody (systemic lupus erythematosus)
Antineutrophil cytoplasmic antibody and complement (vasculitis)
HIV (AIDS)
Hepatitis B serology
ASO (poststrep glomerulonephritis)

Obtain a renal ultrasound to evaluate kidney size.

Nephrotic syndrome
In NS, a glomerular lesion causes loss of protein in the urine.
This leads to proteinuria and hypoalbuminemia. The serum oncotic pressure drops
  and fluid leaks into the tissues, causing edema. The liver attempts to produce more
  protein to compensate for increasing production of lipoproteins and clotting factors,
  leading to hyperlipidemia and hypercoagulability. Urinary immunoglobulin G and M
  (IgG and IgM) loss cause immune deficiency.
Usually presents as a child (especially a male 2 to 7 yrs old) with generalized edema
  (without hypertension); otherwise asymptomatic with the following labs:
  - Proteinuria: >40 mg/hr/m^2; >50 mg/kg/24 hr; Prot:Cr >2.0
  - Hypoalbuminemia: Serum albumin <2.5 g/dL
  - Hypercholesterolemia: Total Chol >200
Minimal change disease (MCD) is the most likely cause. Other idiopathic causes are
  mesangioproliferative and focal segmental glomerular sclerosis.
Immune complex causes such as membranous nephropathy, membranoproliferative
  glomerulonephritis.
There are also secondary causes such as infections (malaria, syphilis), malignancy
  (lymphoma), autoimmune (lupus, Henoch-Schönlein purpura, serum sickness), and
  toxins (heavy metals).

Differential diagnosis
Heart failure: More likely to have rales on lung exam, and urine protein will be negative.
Renal failure: Edema is less likely, and an elevated BUN/Cr is essential.
Cirrhosis: Abdominal/lower extremity swelling, no proteinuria, and no facial/earlobe
  edema.
Benign proteinurias include transient proteinuria and orthostatic proteinuria.

 Refer to the nephrologist
Treat the pt without a biopsy initially as if they had MCD (>75% of cases will be MCD
  and will respond to the therapy). Give prednisone 2 mg/kg (max 75 mg/day) for 4 wks
  with a slow taper over the next 4 wks; 90% of pts will respond in <3 wks.
Even if they respond initially, about 80% will require prednisone off and on over the
  next several years. A relapse is 3 consecutive days of a urine dip with protein of ≥2+.
If they continually relapse, other agents such as cyclophosphamide or cyclosporin can
  be used.
The nephrologist will consider biopsy if the pt fails to respond to immunosuppressants
  or if:
  - There is a strong family history of nephritis or renal failure.
  - There are signs of nephritis, such as hypertension, hematuria, and renal
    insufficiency.

Use furosemide to control edema; add albumin if hemoconcentration causes hematocrit >50%.
Albumin helps prevent intravascular volume depletion during diuresis.

Prevent complications:
Infection: Particularly susceptible to infections from encapsulated organisms such as
  pneumococcus. Give the vaccine and monitor carefully for infection. Treat
  presumptively if the pt arrives with signs of spontaneous bacterial peritonitis:
                    - Ascites   - Abdominal pain   - Fever
Thrombosis: Children with NS are prone to venous thrombosis, so monitor for
  complications such as pulmonary embolus and renal vein thrombosis.

S **Where is the child bleeding from and for how long?**

Nosebleeds are common in children; however, bleeding from both nostrils, the gums, or vaginal and anal mucosae is not.

Cover menstrual histories with all adolescent girls.

Chronic bleeding implies a genetic cause, whereas acute bleeding is consistent with an acquired process.

Does the child also have a rash?

What the parents call a rash may actually be petechiae or purpura.

Does anyone in the family have a problem with bleeding or bruising?

Family history may imply a genetic link.

O **Evaluate the pt's vital signs.**

Tachycardia suggests significant anemia or hypovolemia.

Fever may imply an infectious process, and sepsis should be considered emergently.

Evaluate the pt's color.

Pts with hemoglobins less than 9.0 are generally pale. Good places to check for this are:
- Conjuntiva   - Palate   - Palms of the hands

Look at the mucosae from which the pt has been bleeding.

The nares should be examined for areas of crusted blood that would suggest recent bleeding.

Examine the gingiva for evidence of inflammation suggesting a common gingivitis. Mucosa that is bleeding because of a lack of clotting ability usually will not appear inflamed.

Examine for lymphadenopathy and splenomegaly.

These may imply either a malignant process or an autoimmune phenomenon.

Examine all sites of bruising.

Look for patterns. Bruises that look like household items (electrical cord, belts, etc.) or knuckles may imply child abuse. Bruises of coagulopathy should be patternless.

Look for areas of subcutaneous bleeding.

Petechiae: Small, pinpoint, red, nonblanching macules, which represent subcutaneous capillary bleeding, most commonly appear on the legs, but may also appear on the palate, face, and torso.

Purpura (bruises): Larger nonblanching areas of subcutaneous blood

Perform appropriate labs.

CBC with a differential

PT

PTT

Peripheral smear for examination

A **Idiopathic Thrombocytopenic Purpura (ITP)**
Nosebleeds, gum bleeding, petechiae, and purpura with a very low platelet count. A
high mean platelet volume (MPV) implies autoimmune platelet destruction. Platelets
are larger when they first emerge from the marrow and shrink as they age. Because in
ITP platelets are rapidly destroyed after their release from the bone marrow, the
average platelet is larger than if the platelets were to remain in circulation for their
entire 5- to 7-day life span. All other cell lines on the CBC should be normal.

Differential diagnosis
Leukemia: Thrombocytopenia is accompanied by anemia and/or leukopenia or
leukocytosis. Check for any circulating immature WBC forms (metamyelocytes,
myelocytes, promyelocytes, or blasts). However, even in the absence of these,
leukemia should still be considered, because it can occur with any CBC. It should be
noted, however, that it would be extremely rare for the platelets on a leukemic blood
smear to be large (increased MPV) like those in ITP. It is far more likely that they
would be small or normal sized.
Disseminated intravascular coagulation (DIC): Both PT and PTT are elevated, often
occurring in sepsis. Check the peripheral smear for fragmented RBCs. Without these,
DIC is highly unlikely.
Vitamin K deficiency: An isolated elevated PT that is common in neonates and pts with
chronic intestinal malabsorption.
Hemophilia: An isolated elevated PTT with a lifelong history of muscle and joint bleeds.
Von Willebrand disease: The most common genetic cause of bleeding, it can cause easy
bleeding without the lab findings noted above in hemophilia.
Mucosal infection such as gingivitis, vaginitis, proctitis, etc.
Child abuse: bruising in strange patterns, occult fractures, retinal hemorrhage frenulum
tears.

P **Admit the pt immediately for workup.**
Do not transfuse platelets unless the pt has signs or symptoms of an acute,
life-threatening bleed (e.g., intracranial).
• Giving platelets to a pt who has an autoimmune destruction of platelets may drive
this autoimmunity and cause increased destruction, like adding wood to a fire.

Start intravenous immunoglobulin (IVIG) 1 g/kg over 12 hrs.
IVIG will bind to the Fc receptors on macrophages in the spleen, thus preventing
platelet destruction.

**If suspect or cannot rule out leukemia, a bone marrow biopsy must be
done to diagnose the type of leukemia, or differentiate it from ITP.**
With a diagnosis of leukemia, the bone marrow will be infiltrated with a clonal
population of blast cells, whether they are lymphocytic or myelogenous. Production
of all other cell lines will be decreased.
In ITP, the marrow should appear normal with increased numbers of megakaryocytes
(the cellular precursor to platelets).

**Place the pt on fall precautions because minimal trauma may result in
an intracranial hemorrhage.**
Note that hemorrhage, although a risk, is less likely if the pt has ITP because the young,
large platelets are hyperfunctional and not many are required for clotting.

**If bone marrow biopsy is normal and IVIG ineffective, start prednisone
1–2 mg/kg qd.**
Immunosuppressive steroids should decrease immune activity against platelets.

S **How old is the child?**

The risk of having a severe infection but still appearing well differs by age:
- <28 days of age: High risk
- 29 days to 3 months of age: Moderate risk
- 3 months to 3 yrs of age: Low risk
- >3 yrs of age: Minimal risk

Workup is focused on not missing meningitis or other serious overwhelming infection (sepsis).

If the child is <3 months, it is important to ask about the method of delivery (vaginal or Cesarean section) and if mother was diagnosed with any perinatal infections.

The older the pt, the less likely he or she will be infected by group B streptococcus or herpes simplex, but it is important to note. Neonates are at high risk.

Are there any sick contacts in the home or is the child at day care?

Upper respiratory tract infections (URIs) are highly contagious. Other sick children in the home or at day care may have exposed this child to a common pathogen.

Did the parent take the child's temperature, and if so, how was it taken?

Studies show that parental report of tactile fever usually correlates well with an actual fever.

Rectal temperature is more reliable than axillary. As a general rule, rectal temperature is one degree hotter and axillary temperature is one degree cooler than oral temperature.

O **Check the vitals.**

Even if you have a history of fever, it is still important to document a fever.

Check the oxygen saturation.

A pulse oximetry reading <95% is sensitive for pneumonia in the age group including neonates up through 3 months. All children with low O_2 sats should have a chest x-ray.

Evaluate the child's general appearance.

If the child is well-appearing and comfortable, be reassured.

If the child is irritable and inconsolable by the parents, consider meningitis.

Perform a thorough PE. Look for obvious signs of infection.

Rash: Might indicate viral exanthem, impetigo, or cellulitis.

Rales or rhonchi: On the lung exam, sound like wet Rice Krispies or Velcro, respectively. Suggests atelectasis, fluid overload, or pneumonia.

Bulging fontanelle: Indicates increased intracranial pressure. With fever, consider meningitis.

Oral blisters: Common in a toddler or infant, these are likely to indicate herpangina (back of the oropharynx) or gingival stomatitis (front of the oropharynx).

Erythematous, purulent, enlarged tonsils: Common in children between 5 and 12 yrs of age, streptococcal pharyngitis may be asymptomatic. See Fever with Sore Throat p. 102.

Erythematous, bulging, nonmobile, tympanic membrane suggests otitis media.

Assuming that all of the above indicatory PE findings are negative, what to do next depends, as noted above, on the age group:

Less than or equal to 28 days: CBC with differential, blood culture, urine by in and out catheter for U/A and urine culture, lumbar puncture (LP), sending the cerebrospinal fluid for cell counts, glucose, protein, and culture. No matter the results, the pt will be admitted.

29 days to 3 months: CBC with differential, blood culture, in and out catheter urine for U/A and culture
- *No LP* (per the Rochester Criteria): If U/A is negative, and the WBC is between 5 and 15 without bands.
- *Perform LP:* If the white count is <5 or >15 or there is bandemia, all of which are shown to be indicators of sepsis in this age group.

3 months to 3 yrs: CBC with differential, blood culture, urine by in and out catheter (may cease to do this on males after 1 yr of age) for U/A and culture. Perform LP in this age group only if you see signs suggesting meningitis on PE such as fever with meningismus and/or altered mental status.

Older than 3 yrs: Lab tests only as indicated by PE

A **Fever of unknown etiology. Specific diagnosis differs by age group.**
Rule out sepsis: Less than or equal to 28 days
Fever without source: 29 days to 3 months
Rule out occult bacteremia: 3 months to 3 yrs of age. Usually caused by *Streptococcus pneumoniae* and usually resolves without treatment, but may develop focal infections like meningitis.
More than 3 yrs old: Overwhelming infection is less likely because of mature immune system.

Differential diagnosis
Neuro: Meningitis, encephalitis, spinal abscess
Resp: Pneumonia, bronchitis, tracheitis
CV: Endocarditis
FEN/GI: Salmonellosis, appendicitis
Renal/GU: Cystitis, pyelonephritis
Heme/ID: Leukemia/lymphoma, HIV/TB/Syphilis, any infection

P **<28 days: Admit and observe.**
If the LP results remain negative and the pt develops symptoms of a viral URI, or the fever resolves, no treatment is indicated. May discharge.
If there are indeterminate or (+) LP or CBC results, start vancomycin and cefotaxime IV until the cultures are negative.

29 days to 3 months: If baby is well appearing, CBC is normal, and the parents are reliable, send pt home with a 24-hour recheck. Otherwise admit.
If the LP was done and was negative, give a dose of Rocephin IV or IM and send the pt home with a 24-hour recheck.
If the LP was positive for meningitis, admit and start same regimen as above.

3 months to 3 years and the baby is well appearing:
If the WBC >15, give ceftriaxone and send home with a 24-hour recheck.
If WBC <15, may send home without antibiotics but with a 24-hour recheck.

>3 years old: Reassure the parents. Provide Tylenol (10–15 mg/kg) or ibuprofen (10 mg/kg), but instruct them that fever is a benign entity.
The medication should only be used to alleviate the child's symptoms of fever.

Parents should return child to the hospital if irritable, lethargic, or feeding poorly.

S How old is the child and what symptoms is he or she having?

Nonspecific: Fever, irritability, decreased feeding, vomiting, lethargy

Meningitic symptoms (less common): Bulging fontanelles, seizures

In older children (after about 1 yr), symptoms of meningitis include headache, neck stiffness, spontaneous vomiting, photophobia, seizures, altered mental status (AMS), focal neurologic deficits, and lethargy.

O Carefully examine the child, looking for signs of meningitis and source of the fever.

Vitals: Fever and tachycardia are likely. Hypotension is an ominous sign.

AMS: Confusion, lethargy, somnolence, coma

Stiff neck: Ask pt to touch chin to chest.

- Brudzinski's sign is positive if on passive neck flexion the knees bend or there is leg pain.
- Kernig's sign: Flex the hip 90 degrees and try to straighten leg at knee; test + if unable to straighten leg.

Skin lesions: Petechiae (small, nonblanching red spots) and purpura (coalesced spots into bruises) may indicate a fulminant infection, such as one with meningococcus.

Look for any site from which a bacterial infection could have invaded into the meninges:

- *Sinusitis:* Facial tenderness and halitosis
- *Otitis media:* Bulging, erythematous tympanic membrane
- *Mastoiditis:* Postauricular swelling that pushes the pinna forward

Obtain appropriate labs and studies.

CBC with differential and blood culture. Indications of a bacterial infection include elevated WBC, neutrophilia, and bandemia.

Obtain U/A and urine culture to rule out urinary tract infection, also a possible diagnosis.

Deciding to perform a lumbar puncture (LP).

If you suspect meningitis, it is imperative that you perform an LP. Contraindications include failure to obtain informed consent from the parents and signs of increased intracranial pressure (ICP), such as bulging fontanelle, papilledema, and focal neurologic deficits.

If you suspect increased ICP, obtain a head CT to assess ventricular patency.

Interpreting the LP results.

Check opening pressure in older children. Normal is 15 to 22 cm H_2O.

Color: Yellow cerebrospinal fluid (CSF) is called xanthochromia (breaking down RBCs turns the CSF yellow, suggesting their long-term presence). Cloudy CSF suggests infection.

Tube 1: Send for a culture and Gram stain.

Tube 2: Send for protein and glucose levels. Protein is normally between 15 and 50. A protein >50 is the most consistent sign of an abnormal LP. Normal glucose is about two-thirds of the serum glucose (~60–80). In bacterial meningitis, it is likely to be low.

Tube 3: Send for cell count. This will give you:

- RBCs: Vary (0–1000s) depending on how traumatic the LP was. However, the presence of xanthochromia may indicate herpes or subarachnoid hemorrhage.
- WBCs: Normal is <20 in newborns, <8 in older pts. Add ~1 WBC per 500 RBCs.
- Differential: Predominant cell type is a clue as to the type of infection.

Tube 4: Save this tube for any *special tests* indicated by history, exam, or the results from the other three tubes. Special tests include tuberculosis (TB) culture, viral polymerase chain reaction, and India ink for fungus.

Meningitis. Etiologies include:
Neonates (<28 days old): Group B strep, *E. coli*, *Listeria monocytogenes*
Older children: *S. pneumoniae* and *N. meningitides*. *Haemophilus influenzae* type
 B used to be a common and life-threatening cause, but it is extremely rare since the
 advent of the vaccine.
Viral meningitis is a possibility in all age groups. Enterovirus is the most common
 pathogen, and it occurs most frequently in the summer. It is essentially benign.
A history of TB exposure should be present to make a diagnosis of TB meningitis. It
 can cause meningeal obstruction and often fatal hydrocephalus.

Before performing an LP, consider the differential diagnosis:
Acute enteritis: Fever and vomiting followed by diarrhea within 8 hrs
Urinary tract infection: Can cause fever and vomiting but not irritability
Pneumonia: Usually a cough will be present. Check a chest x-ray.
Subarachnoid hemorrhage: Blood in the CSF causes meningeal inflammation.
 Symptoms may mimic meningitis. Fever and head CT should help differentiate the
 two.
Now perform the LP and put all of the CSF clues together (Table 6).

Table 6					
Infection	**WBC**	**Diff**	**Glucose**	**Protein**	**Color**
Preemie	<16	Normal	60–80	15–120	Clear
Normal	<8	Normal	60–80	15–50	Clear
Bacterial	>500	PMNs	0–20	>100	Cloudy
Partially Txd	>500	Variable	20–40	>100	Variable
Viral	>10	Lymphs	60–80	50–150	Usually clear
Herpes	>10	Lymphs	60–80	50-150	Bloody, xanthochromic
TB	20–200	Lymphs	0–10	200–2 g	Usually cloudy

P **Admit this pt for treatment. For suspected bacterial meningitides,
consider an ICU admission. Initiate treatment in the ER.**
For possible bacterial infections:
   • In preemies, start ampicillin, cefotaxime, and vancomycin.
   • In neonates, start ampicillin and cefotaxime +/− dexamethasone.
   • In children, start cefotaxime, vancomycin, and dexamethasone.
If you suspect herpes, start acyclovir IV, continue for 21 days if workup +.
For possible fungal, TB, or other chronic infections, start antibiotics and await
 confirmation of diagnosis before treatment unless high clinical suspicion and the pt is
 unstable.

**As always with sick pts, IV fluids and respiratory support are mainstays
of treatment.**

S

Is there fever and productive cough?
A temperature over 101.3°F with a productive or productive-sounding cough of abrupt onset is most typical for pneumonia. Shortness of breath and tachypnea are also common.

How long has this been going on?
If the cough is chronic or without fever, consider alternative diagnoses such as asthma or pertussis.

Does the child have any underlying diseases, which may place him or her at higher risk for certain types of pneumonias?
Cystic fibrosis: Staphylococcal and *Pseudomonas* infections become more likely.
Asthma: CAP and atypical pneumonias
Sickle cell disease: Consider acute chest syndrome.
AIDS: Consider *Pneumocystis carinii* pneumonia, cytomegalovirus, or fungus.
Neurologic impairment: Such as cerebral palsy, be suspicious for aspiration pneumonia.

Where is the child from and has the child traveled anywhere recently?
American Southwest: Consider coccidioidomycosis and, although unlikely, Hantavirus.
American Midwest: Consider histoplasmosis or blastomycosis.
Developing countries: Consider salmonella, measles, and tuberculosis.

O

Examine pt.
Do standard exam with emphasis on the lung fields.

Look for signs of respiratory distress.
Look for poor air movement, use of accessory muscles of respiration, or tachypnea.

Listen to lungs for any focal area of sound change.
- Wheeze (high-pitched, almost whistle-like)   - Decreased air movement
- Rhonchi (course, Velcro-like breath sounds)   - Crackles (fine Rice Krispies like sounds)

Percuss lung fields for any signs of consolidation.
If there is dullness, consider effusion or infiltrate. Tympany, a loud, hollow sound, suggests pneumothorax or obstructive disease such as asthma. If you have difficulty interpreting percussion, consider performing:
- Whispered pectoriloquy (pt whisper syllables such as 'A' while you listen and auscultate the lung fields)
- Tactile fremitus (pt says "ninety-nine" while you palpate the chest and back)

In both of the above exams, increased transmission of the sound occurs with pulmonary consolidation, as in pneumonia, and decreased transmission occurs with free air (pneumothorax) or obstructive disease (e.g., asthma).

Obtain a chest x-ray (CXR).
Look for signs of consolidation or effusion.

A

Pneumonia
Inflammation of the lungs with infiltrate on CXR

Pneumonia can be broken down into three main types:
Community-acquired pneumonia (CAP)
- *Lobar pneumonia:* As the name suggests, an entire lobe or part of a lobe is filled with pus and appears white on CXR. Most common etiology is *Streptococcus pneumoniae*, but *Haemophilus influenzae* and *Klebsiella pneumoniae* are also common.
- *Atypical pneumonia:* Characterized by hazy bilateral or patchy interstitial infiltrates on the CXR. Typical etiologies are *Mycoplasma pneumoniae, Chlamydia pneumoniae*, or *psittaci*. Common in adolescents and can be accompanied by rashes or joint pain.
- *Viral pneumonia:* Can look like either of the two above, but usually causes minimal infiltrates. Common etiologies are influenza, respiratory syncytial virus, and adenovirus.

Nosocomial (hospital-acquired) pneumonia: Consider *Pseudomonas aeruginosa, Staphylococcus aureus*, or whatever bacterial outbreak is occurring in your institution.
Aspiration pneumonia: If the pt is neurologically or developmentally impaired, *Staphylococcus aureus* and anaerobic organisms are most common.

Differential diagnosis
Even if there is an infiltrate on the CXR, you should consider any one of the following not only as possible alternatives to your diagnosis but also as possible comorbid conditions.
- *Asthma:* Chronic cough, worse at night, wheezing, chest tightness, shortness of breath
- *Acute bronchitis:* May have the white count and infection symptoms, but lack an infiltrate on CXR. *Haemophilus influenzae* is the most likely etiology.
- *Viral upper respiratory infection (URI):* Milder symptoms including nasal and pharyngeal complaints.
- *Pertussis:* Chronic cough, paroxysmal cough, post-tussive emesis, whoop (if older than 6 months), and URI symptoms.
- Consider immunodeficiency or cystic fibrosis (regardless of race) if the pt has had multiple/frequent pneumonias.

P

<30 days old, admit and treat with ampicillin 100 mg/kg/day divided q6h and cefotaxime 100 mg/kg/day divided q6h.
Admit any baby less than 30 days old with a fever.
Likely bacteria are Group B strep, *E. coli, Listeria, Strep pneumo, H. influenzae*.

>30 days old, treat with ampicillin/sulbactam 200 mg/kg/day divided q6h IV, then when pt improves, amoxicillin/clavulanate 40 mg/kg/day divided q8h to finish 10-day course.
Likely bacteria are *Strep pneumo, Staph aureus, Moraxella, H. influenza, and Neisseria meningitidis.*

If you suspect an atypical pneumonia such as mycoplasma or *C. pneumoniae*, consider azithromycin 10 mg/kg (max 500 mg) on first day and then half of that dose for the next 4 days.

Admit for:
Any signs of respiratory distress or unstable vital signs
Persistent oxygen requirement

S   **What is the time course of the symptoms? Are there any associated symptoms?**
Typically, croup starts with a low-grade fever and a mild runny nose for up to a week, followed by hoarseness, fever, and a barking cough or stridor. Pts usually present on the second or third day of the illness.

Is there any change in the stridor with position change?
If the stridor (hoarse cough) changes with position, consider foreign body.

Is the child toxic-appearing or drooling?
If the child is toxic-appearing (looks extremely sick and very tired), and especially if the child has been drooling in tripod position, consider epiglottitis.

Is the cough productive or dry?
Productive coughs tend to be intrapulmonary processes, whereas dry coughs tend to be intrapulmonary or upper airway.

Have the parents noticed any signs of respiratory distress?
- Unable to speak in   - Tachypnea
  full sentences   - Suprasternal retractions
- Accessory respiratory   - Abdominal breathing
  muscle usage   - Nasal flaring
- Subcostal retractions

How old is the child?
Croup can occur at any age but usually occurs between 3 months and 3 yrs.

O   **Evaluate the vital signs and pulse-ox.**
Expect a low-grade fever, although high fever does not rule out croup. Lack of fever may indicate a foreign body aspiration.
Be concerned about a child with tachypnea and tachycardia.
Be *very* concerned about a child with slow respirations or bradycardia.
Pulse-ox should be greater than or equal to 95% on room air.

Observe and listen to the child from the door (being careful not to agitate the child). What do you see and hear?
Note the mental status of the pt, which can range from agitation to obtundation.
Notice the child's color for any signs of cyanosis.
Auscultate, looking for decreased air movement.
Assess work of breathing by looking for signs of respiratory distress such as subcostal, intracostal, and supraclavicular retractions, and nasal flaring.
Listen for an intermittent barking cough that sounds similar to the sound produced by a seal.
Listen closely for stridor. Stridor at rest is a worrisome sign.

If the diagnosis is uncertain, obtain a posteroanterior (PA) chest and lateral neck x-rays.
Croup will display a narrowing of the subglottic airway on PA chest x-ray with some local haziness. The lateral neck films will help rule out epiglottitis and retropharyngeal abscess.

Acute Laryngotracheobronchitis or Croup

An acute subglottic inflammatory process (the narrowing of the area below the glottis causes the stridor), which is almost always viral in nature. Parainfluenza (types 1–3) causes most of the cases. Influenza, adenovirus, respiratory syncytial virus, and measles are less common causes.

Assess the degree of stridor and of respiratory distress.

If the pt has stridor at rest, poor air movement, cyanosis, severe retractions, and/or tachypnea to a significant degree, or worse, tiring out and obtundation, monitor carefully and watch for possible respiratory failure.

Differential diagnosis

Carefully consider and rule out:
- *Foreign body aspiration:* Afebrile
- *Epiglottitis:* Toxic-appearing, febrile, no cough, drooling
- *Retropharyngeal abscess:* Dysphagia, neck stiffness
- *Bacterial tracheitis:* Toxic, copious tracheal secretions
- *Acute asthma exacerbation:* Cough, wheezing, no stridor
- *Spasmodic croup:* Spontaneous resolution

P **Initial treatment is always cool mist for 20 to 30 minutes.**

The aim of all therapy is to shrink the edema (increase the size of the airway). Cold, humidified air induces local vasoconstriction. Have the parent hold the mask slightly away from the child's face, again so as not to agitate the child.

Add oxygen to the mist, 4 L/min of flow. Follow the pulse-ox.

If the pulse-ox is less than 95%:

Start epinephrine 1:1000.

If the pt has stridor at rest, or stridor persists after cool mist:

Racemic Epi 0.5 cc in 3 cc normal saline can also be used, but there is no difference in effect and it is more expensive.

Epi acts at the subglottic inflammation with direct α_1 agonist properties to induce local vasoconstriction.

Administer dexamethasone (a corticosteroid) 0.6 mg/kg.

If the pt has moderate to severe croup, but responds to cool mist.

Significantly decreases inflammation for several hours and prevents late phase of allergic reaction.

Parental advice on discharge:

Most children with croup do not need to be admitted, and it will usually resolve spontaneously within 3 to 5 days.

Admit for:

Persistent signs of respiratory distress despite treatment or suspicion of tracheitis, epiglottitis, retropharyngeal abscess, or foreign body.

S **How old is the child?**

Bronchiolitis is an inflammatory obstruction of the small airways, usually caused by respiratory syncytial virus (RSV). Other possible etiologies are:

- Parainfluenza virus   - Mycoplasma
- Adenoviruses   - Other viruses

Bronchiolitis tends to occur in children younger than 2 yrs of age, with most cases occurring between 3 to 6 months. If child is older than 2 yrs, consider an alternative diagnosis.

What time of year is it?

Bronchiolitis usually occurs between December and June.

Is anyone else at home sick?

Often, someone else at home will have upper respiratory infection (URI) symptoms. The disease is much milder in older hosts because they have larger-diameter airways and a more mature immune system.

Is the child male, bottle-fed, attending day care, around a smoker, or in a crowded home?

These are all risk factors for bronchiolitis.

What are the child's symptoms?

RSV usually begins with runny nose, sneezing, and low-grade fever, and progresses after 1 to 3 days to a paroxysmal wheezy cough and eventually shortness of breath and respiratory distress. If there are other systemic symptoms, such as vomiting or diarrhea, consider alternative diagnoses.

O **Perform a PE.**

Listen to the lungs carefully for rhonchi, crackles, and wheezing.

Look carefully for signs of respiratory distress:

- Accessory respiratory muscle usage   - Tachypnea
- Tachycardia   - Cyanosis
- Nasal flaring   - Suprasternal retractions
- Subcostal retractions   - Abdominal breathing

If disease progresses enough, may have poor air movement followed by lethargy and apnea.

Liver may be palpable as a result of lung hyperinflation.

Pulse oximeter

Often the oxygen saturation will be less than 94%.

Arterial blood gas

It will commonly show hypoxia, hypercapnia, and acidosis.

Chest x-ray

Initially it will be normal. Some will have:

- Hyperexpansion   - Peribronchial cuffing   - Segmental consolidation

Swab the nasopharynx and send for an RSV enzyme-linked immunoassay or culture.

To confirm, not rule out, the diagnosis. A negative test only means RSV was missed or another virus is responsible.

There are epidemiologic factors to consider here as well. It is important to know when the first case of RSV arrives in your hospital every winter.

A **Bronchiolitis**

A viral infection of the small airways leading to inflammation and obstructive asthma-like symptoms, including wheezing and hyperexpansion. Because resistance to flow in a tube is inversely proportional to the radius to the 4th power, and only young children have such small airways, this usually only occurs in children younger than 2 yrs old. After this, airways are too large for simple inflammation to incur sufficient change to laminar airflow.

RSV is the most common etiology; others include influenza, parainfluenza, and adenovirus.

Differential diagnosis

Asthma: Especially if there is a family history of asthma, repeated episodes of bronchiolitis, sudden onset of URI symptoms without a prodrome, or good response to a single dose of albuterol. There is unlikely to be a fever.

Chronic aspiration caused by tracheoesophageal fistula or neurologic deficit: Consider if respiratory difficulty occurred with feeds preceding the recent episode.

Cystic fibrosis: Frequent/chronic pneumonias. Check sweat chloride.

Laryngotracheomalacia: History of prematurity with intubation or stridor since birth.

Bronchopulmonary dysplasia: History of prematurity with intubation and chronic wheeze.

Heart failure: See Heart Failure p. 20.

Tracheal or bronchial foreign body: Sudden onset, no prodrome, a lack of fever, and unilateral breath sounds should make you consider this diagnosis.

Pertussis: Pt looks well between paroxysmal coughing jags; also, the prodrome is longer.

Bacterial bronchopneumonia: Poor response to just supportive measures, infiltrate on chest x-ray (CXR).

Chlamydia trachomatis pneumonia: Affects children 1 to 4 months old with more cough and less wheezing or fever. There are usually patchy infiltrates bilaterally on the CXR.

 P **Give humidified oxygen.**

Moist air lubricates mucus and the oxygen can penetrate to the alveoli.

Racemic epinephrine by handheld nebulizer is not shown to be effective but still is often used.

Positioning the infant with the head of the bed slightly elevated and with the neck slightly extended (sniffing position)

This will improve air entry.

Give IV fluids at about 1.5 times maintenance rate.

Hydration will increase clearance of respiratory secretions.

Oral feeding may risk respiratory distress. Consider nasogastric feedings also.

If interstitial pneumonia on CXR, consider starting a macrolide antibiotic.

This will cover atypical organisms such as *Mycoplasma* and *Chlamydia*.

Admit:

If supplemental oxygen is required to maintain oxygen saturation.

If the pt cannot tolerate feeds because of respiratory difficulty.

If there are signs of respiratory distress.

Consider bilevel positive airway pressure or intubation with mechanical ventilation if respiratory distress worsens despite aggressive treatment.

This will merit transfer to the ICU.

S **Has the child had any fever?**
(+) fever suggests infection: Pneumonia, sinusitis, otitis media
(−) fever suggests noninfectious etiology: Asthma, foreign body

Is the child behaving normally?
If the child is lethargic, toxic (extremely ill) appearing, or obtunded, these are all signs
that the child may have more than just the common cold (URI).
If the child has a fever, cough, and runny nose, but is otherwise behaving normally and
playing, this is probably only a viral URI and nothing needs to be done.

What are the associated symptoms?
Ask if there are any symptoms (run through your review of systems) to see if anything
would lead you to believe:
- Common cold: Cough, rhinitis, sore throat
- More than just a cold: Ear pain, drooling, shortness of breath, bad breath,
  vomiting, voice change

O **Evaluate the vital signs.**
Although children can commonly have fevers to any degree, a low-grade fever (less
than 102.5°F) is more indicative of a rhinoviral infection.
Mild tachycardia may be present with fever, but tachypnea would be unusual.

Assess the general appearance of the child.
The child should appear nontoxic because these URIs are rarely severe. Signs of
respiratory distress, such as retractions and nasal flaring, should not be present.

Perform an exam of the eyes, nose, ears, throat, and lungs.
Eyes: Red eyes with swollen conjunctiva likely indicate conjunctivitis, which is common
in toddlers who rub nasal secretions into their eyes. It will usually be bilateral with
scant discharge. A unilateral, markedly red eye with gross purulent discharge suggests
bacterial conjunctivitis.
Nose: Nasal passages should be red, swollen, congested, and full of mucus ranging in
color from clear to green. Pale, boggy-appearing mucosa suggests allergic rhinitis.
Ears: Tympanic membranes should be nonerythematous, with normal landmarks and
light reflex (cone-shaped reflection of the light on the anterior inferior quadrant). A
bulging, red eardrum, with distortion of the normal landmarks or light reflex with
decreased movement to insufflation suggests an acute otitis media.
Mouth and throat: May appear mildly red, but the tonsils should not be red or have any
pus on them if they are visible at all. There should be no lesions on the roof of the
mouth.
Lungs: Despite the cough, the lungs should sound clear with good air movement. Extra
sounds such as the following should prompt further workup of a pulmonary process
such as pneumonia or asthma:
- Wheezing: Expiratory whistling high-pitched noises
- Rhonchi: A harsh sound like the one made by Velcro
- Rales: Crackles like the sounds made by wet Rice Krispies
Percuss the lung for dullness. If it is found, check to see if the area of dullness transmits
sound through either egophony or tactile fremitus. If the dullness transmits sound,
then it is a consolidation; if not, it is an effusion (collection of liquid).

A Viral Upper Respiratory Tract Infection (URI)

This is the most minor form of infection and one of the most common reasons for pediatric ER visits. It is characterized by involvement of the eyes, nose, and throat with minor symptoms in each area. The most common bacterial complications of these illnesses are:

- *Otitis media:* Characterized by a red, bulging tympanic membrane with decreased movement to insufflation. In children who are old enough to express it, there should be reported pain. Common pathogens are *Streptococcus pneumoniae, Haemophilus influenzae,* and *Moraxella catarrhalis.* Mastoiditis, characterized by mastoid pain and anterior displacement of the pinna, is a rare complication.
- *Sinusitis:* Occurs when the small meatus that drains the sinuses become obstructed for prolonged periods by inflamed nasal mucosa. Should be considered any time a viral URI continues to have fever for longer than 1 week. Characterized by tenderness to palpation of the forehead over the eyes or of the cheekbones, postnasal drip, and halitosis.

Differential diagnosis

The H&P should rapidly rule out the following more serious infections:

- Pharyngitis   - Epiglottitis   - Meningitis   - Pneumonia   - Sepsis

P If the pt lacks evidence of a bacterial process or complication, reassure the parents.

Antibiotics are only for bacterial infections, so in the case of viral URIs or colds, they are completely useless. As a result, the benefits of taking the medicines do not outweigh the risks of adverse reactions and developing microbial resistance, so antibiotics should not be used.

Fever control: Many parents are only in the ER because of fever. Reassure the parents that fever is a benign condition that cannot harm their child. Fever is only the body's reaction to infection. The infection, not the fever, can be dangerous, but if you are comfortable that it is a viral URI, then the fever poses no risk. To make the pt more comfortable, acetaminophen or ibuprofen can be given.

Cough suppressant: Many parents want to stop their child from coughing, but coughing clears the airway. In the end, it is beneficial to the pt. If the parents insist, any guifenasin-dextramethorphan combination at bedtime will suffice to suppress coughing.

If otitis media is present, start amoxicillin, 15 mg/kg/dose tid for 10 days.

Most children get better without antibiotics, but if you diagnose acute otitis media, standard practice is to treat. If the fever persists after 7 days, switch to amoxicillin with clavulanate.

If sinusitis is suspected, give the same dose of amoxicillin, but continue for 14 days.

Antibiotic penetration of obstructed sinuses is difficult, so longer therapy is necessary.

There are no admission criteria for these illnesses unless you suspect sepsis or meningitis.

How old is the child?

Different age ranges represent increased risk of different pharyngitides:
- Infants and toddlers are at risk for herpangina. These pts have blisters on their tonsillar pillars and often high fever. The blisters are painful, so the pts will not want to eat.
- 5 to 15 yrs old is the usual range for strep throat (streptococcal pharyngitis), but it can occur at any age. It is extremely uncommon before 2 yrs and less severe after 20 yrs old.
- From 15 years through adolescence and young adulthood, mono (mononucleosis) is a common cause of pharyngitis.

What symptoms is the child having?

Common symptoms associated with pharyngitis (sore throat) are:
- Headache   - Abdominal pain   - +/− Nausea/Vomiting
- Fever   - +/− Dysphagia   - Cough   - Rhinorrhea

One way to differentiate strep throat from other upper respiratory infections (URIs) is that cough and rhinorrhea are usually not present in strep throat.

Examine the throat.

There are many different ways a sore throat can appear on PE:
- *Herpangina* (caused by coxsackievirus): Generalized redness with painful ulcers toward the back of the mouth (tonsillar pillars and soft palate)
- *Herpes simplex virus I* (HSV-1 usually occurs around the mouth and HSV-2 usually occurs around the genitalia, but both can do both): Causes ulcerations more anterior in the mouth (gingiva, lips, and tongue).
- Both strep throat and mono present as exudative pharyngitis: Beefy redness restricted to the pharynx, with enlarged tonsils, with or without the presence of pus.
- Peritonsillar abscess presents as unilateral tonsillar enlargement and uvular deviation, especially if associated with a muffled voice.

Finish a general PE, looking for these other common signs:

Scarlatiniform rash (scarlet fever) is a velvety or sandpaper-like rash with Pastia's lines and circumoral pallor; diagnostic of strep.

Tender anterior cervical lymphadenopathy is common in all of these illnesses.

Blisters on the hands and feet are common with coxsackie infections (hand, foot, and mouth disease).

Splenomegaly is associated with infectious mono.

Prominent cough, rhinorrhea, or otitis media make strep throat, mono, and herpangina less likely.

Perform necessary lab tests:

Rapid strep test and throat culture.

Monospot and Epstein-Barr virus (EBV) titers. CBC with differential should show lymphocytosis with atypical lymphocytes in mono.

A **Pharyngitis**
Caused by infectious inflammation of the throat or pharynx.

Differential diagnosis
Strep throat caused by Group A strep or *Streptococcus pyogenes*. Scarlet fever is
associated with a toxin-producing strain.

Strep throat diagnosis mnemonic: A PUFL MN (a puffle man); the more of these
criteria that are positive, the more likely it is to be strep throat:
- *Age* (5–15 yrs)
- *Ø URI* symptoms (no cough/ rhinorrhea)
- *Lympadenopathy* (tender cervical)
- *Pharyngitis* (w/beefy red tonsils)
- *Fever*
- *May to November* (peak incidence)

Herpangina, and hand, foot and mouth disease are caused by coxsackieviruses and can
be diagnosed by the ulcers located posteriorly in the mouth and pharynx.

Herpes stomatitis (usually HSV-1) causes ulcers in the more anterior portion of the
mouth.

Mononucleosis is a syndrome usually caused by EBV. It is characterized by exudative
pharyngitis, low-grade fevers, fatigue, lymphocytosis, and splenomegaly.

Interpret the rapid strep and throat culture.
Diagnostic if the rapid strep or throat culture is positive.

If the rapid strep is negative, you may wait for the throat culture results to treat, or you
may treat immediately if your clinical suspicion for strep throat is high (more of the
above criteria = remember A PUFL MN).

If the throat culture is positive, either start or continue treatment.

If throat culture is negative, remember that some false negatives exist and continue to
treat if your clinical suspicion remains high.

Rule out strep throat to avoid its complications and sequelae.
Treating strep throat reduces incidence of complications such as peritonsillar abscess
and cervical lymphadenitis and sequelae such as rheumatic fever (responsible for
irreversible heart valve lesions) and glomerulonephritis. Initiate therapy within 9 days
of the onset of symptoms to prevent rheumatic fever.

P **Treatment with penicillin V-K 15 mg/kg (max 500 mg) tid for 10 days
(treatment of choice)**
Although bacterial resistance has emerged as a problem with other bacteria worldwide,
Group A Strep remains remarkably sensitive to penicillin. It will continue to be the
drug of choice until resistance is more commonly seen.

If the pt is allergic to penicillin, treat with azithromycin.
Azithromycin can be given but is considerably more expensive. In addition, resistance
develops rapidly, so it should be reserved only for those pts who are truly allergic to
penicillin.

Herpangina and mono are viral illnesses requiring only supportive care.
Children with herpangina should be encouraged to take cool liquids to avoid
dehydration.

Adolescents with mono should get plenty of rest and refrain from kissing and sharing
glasses or cans of soda.

S   **Obtain a general history of the complaint.**
Urinary tract infections (UTIs) can present in almost any age group in many different ways.
- It can present as simple dysuria without fever; usually described as a burning with urination, frequent urinations with minimal urine produced, and a generalized discomfort.
- UTIs can also present with just fever, especially in the neonatal and infancy periods.

Culture urine when the pt has fever and no source (see Fever Without Associated Symptoms p. 90).

Does it burn when the pt urinates?
(Dysuria) This is one of the most common symptoms of UTI.

Is the pt waking up at night to urinate or having small, frequent urinations?
Urinary frequency is another symptom of UTI, and nocturia is a good way of assessing it because children usually do not wake up more than once or twice, if at all, to go to the bathroom at night.

Does the pt have any associated symptoms?
Flank pain is associated with pyelonephritis (infection that has ascended to the kidneys).
Vomiting is common in UTIs in infants. In older children, it is likely to indicate pyelonephritis.
Pyelonephritis is also associated with higher fevers and chills.
Severe abdominal pain when the pt cannot hold still may indicate an associated renal stone. This is the opposite of what is seen in appendicitis, where pts try to hold very still.

Has the pt had UTIs before? If so, how many and how often?
Multiple UTIs suggests a urinary tract abnormality, poor hygiene, or possible sexual abuse.

If pt is a female child, how does she wipe herself?
Wiping back to front is a risk for UTIs.

Is pt sexually active?
Sexually active females have an increased risk for UTIs.

O   **Evaluate the pt's general appearance and vital signs.**
Pt may appear uncomfortable, but should not appear ill or toxic. Mental status and BP should be normal, and the pt should not be tachycardic unless febrile or in pain.

Pt's age and sex
Infants are at high risk for UTIs (males more than females).
Males: 6 months to 1 year old, the risk of a UTI in anatomically normal males drops to almost zero. UTI symptoms in adolescent boys is more commonly sexually transmitted infections.
Females: The risk of UTI in females peaks from 6 months to 2 yrs old and then again in adolescence.

Perform a focused and directed PE.
Check for costovertebral angle (CVA) tenderness on the flank at about the 10th through 12th ribs (pyelonephritis).
Tenderness just above the pubic symphysis is suprapubic tenderness suggestive of cystitis.
Look for lesions and discharge on genital exam.

Obtain a urine sample.

Perform in-and-out catheterization for young children. Bag specimen (sealing a bag over the genitalia) is not useful for culture to rule out UTI because of frequent contamination.

In children who are toilet trained, obtain a clean-catch specimen. Have the pt clean the genital area with several moist sterile towelettes, let the first portion of urine go into the toilet, and then catch the middle portion in the specimen cup.

Obtain a U/A (dipstick or lab) and send a specimen for culture.

Positive nitrite and leukocyte esterase indicate UTI. Bacteria produce nitrites while sitting in the bladder, and white cells produce leukocyte esterase. Very young infants hold almost no urine in their bladders, so these tests are less sensitive. This is why a culture is also necessary.

Microscopic blood can be caused by UTI but not without a positive nitrite or leukocyte esterase.

Positive glucose suggests diabetes mellitus, a risk factor for pyelonephritis at any age.

Urinary Tract Infection

Infections range from a simple cystitis (bacteria growing in the bladder) to a pyelonephritis (bacterial infection of the kidney). Pyelonephritis is more common with anatomic abnormalities of the urinary tract but can occur in completely normal hosts.

Differential diagnosis

The differential of the main features of cystitis are:
- *Dysuria:* Trauma, chemical irritant, stricture, foreign body
- *Frequency:* Diabetic ketoacidosis, polydypsia, microbladder
- *Suprapubic tenderness:* Trauma, tumor, appendicitis
- *Fever:* Sepsis, bacteremia, meningitis

The differential of the features of pyelonephritis are:
- *CVA tenderness:* Appendicitis, trauma, renal colic
- *Vomiting:* Central nervous system (CNS) abnormality, CNS bleed, enteritis

P
Treat with trimethoprim-sulfamethoxazole (TMP-SMX) bid for 7 days.

If TMP-SMX is ineffective, try amoxicillin or cephalexin.

Admit all pts less than 2 months of age for urosepsis. Admit all pts with pyelonephritis who are not tolerating oral intake for IV antibiotics.

At less than 2 months old, it is difficult to contain infection, so the pt is more likely to develop sepsis.

Females more than 5 yrs old and all males, and any pts who are now having a repeat episode of pyelonephritis, require a workup for urinary tract abnormalities.

Repeat urine culture: 3 days into their treatment.

VCUG: After a negative culture, the pt may have a vesiculocystourethrogram (VCUG), which will reveal most abnormalities, such as ureteral reflux and posterior urethral valve.

Renal U/S: To rule out hydronephrosis, scarring, or dysplasia.

Start prophylactic antibiotics (usually Keflex or Bactrim) on any child with a urologic abnormality such as posterior urethral valves and then refer to Urology.

S   **How long has the child had the rash?**
Time course of the rash may help in the diagnosis of the illness.

How long has the child had fever, and what relation does it have to the rash?
Fever usually precedes a rash. Most rashes that coexist with fever are secondary to viral illnesses. Therefore, many of them have a prodrome of fever.
A high fever (greater than 104°F) for 5 days or more preceding the rash should make you suspicious of Kawasaki disease (see Kawasaki Disease p. 110).

Does the pt have any associated symptoms?
Scarlet fever: Sore throat (streptococcal pharyngitis) with sandpaper rash and Pastia's lines
Rheumatic fever: J♥NES is a good mnemonic:
      - Joints: migratory polyarthritis - ♥ Carditis   - Nodules (subcutaneous)
      - Erythema marginatum: Pink macules coalesce into serpiginous pattern
      - Sydenham's chorea

Meningococcemia: This is an emergency. Headache, purpuric rash on legs, photophobia, altered mental status (AMS), vomiting
Epstein-Barr virus (EBV, mononucleosis): Fatigue, lymphadenopathy, sore throat
Measles: Cough, conjunctivitis, coryza (runny nose)
Erythema multiforme may be associated with cough because mycoplasma is a common etiology.
Viral gastroenteritis: Can occasionally develop a rash.

Is the child taking any medications?
Many medications can cause a rash and fever as an allergic reaction. Mononucleosis causes a salmon-pink rash on the trunk in response to amoxicillin or ampicillin.

What is the distribution of the rash?
The pattern or distribution of the rash can help form your differential diagnosis.

Has the child had all of his or her vaccinations? Ask to see the card documenting this.
An up-to-date vaccine card would not rule out measles, rubella, and varicella (all common viral causes of rashes), but they become far less likely.

O   **Evaluate pt's general appearance.**
It is important to note when the pt is "toxic" appearing:
      - Extremely ill   - Poor spontaneous activity   - Pallor
      - Irritability   - AMS
With fever and rash this would suggest sepsis, meningococcemia, or some other dangerous condition and learning to recognize the difference is extremely important.

Describe the rash. Be sure to use gloves while touching lesions.
The rash should be characterized regarding its location on the body, as noted above, and if it forms any patterns, such as sun-exposed areas.
The rash should also be characterized by lesion type (Table 7):
Nodules are dermal (deeper), whereas papules/plaques are epidermal (shallow).

A   **Viral Exanthem**
Erythema infectiosum (fifth disease): Etiology is Parvovirus B_{19}.
- Red rash on each cheek (a slapped-cheek appearance)
- Followed by generalized red maculopapular rash, which becomes lacy in appearance

Table 7 Lesion Types				
Lesion	Flat	Round, Raised	Nonblanching	Fluid-Filled
<5 mm	Macules	Papules	Petechiae	Vesicle
>5 mm	Patches	Plaque	Purpura	Bullae

Varicella (chicken pox): Etiology is varicella-zoster virus
  - Highly contagious   - Generalized distribution   - Pruritic
  - Three different lesions: pink papule, vesicle (dewdrop on a rose petal), and scabbing ulceration. All three lesions should be seen on a pt at once.
Roseola infantum (exanthem subitum, sixth disease): Etiology is human herpes virus 6.
  - High fever, 2–3 days   - Well-appearing child   - Febrile seizure common
  - Fever followed by erythematous rash with small macules and papules surrounded by a pale ring appears. Distribution is usually on the neck, trunk, and behind the ears.
Measles (rubeola): Etiology is a paramyxovirus, rare since vaccine.
  • Prodrome is triad: Cough, coryza, conjunctivitis.
  • Rash is red, maculopapular, starts on the forehead and ears, then spreads over body.
  • Koplik's spots present on the buccal mucosa immediately preceding rash.

Differential diagnosis
Scarlet fever: Etiology is complication of Group A Strep (GAS) pharyngitis.
  • Red, sandpaper-like (small papules), generalized, with Pastia's lines in the flexion creases.
Rheumatic fever: Sequelae of GAS infection; see Jones Criteria above.
Impetigo: A localized streptococcal or staphylococcal skin infection
          - Localized to face   - Macules become vesicles   →   - Honey-crusting
          or extremities
Cellulitis: A spreading streptococcal or staphylococcal skin infection
          - Violaceously red, swollen, hot to the touch   - Usually on the limbs
Meningococcemia: A systemic infection caused by *Neisseria meningitides*
  • Purpura fulminans (most severe form): Complicated by disseminated intravascular coagulation, causing petechiae and ecchymoses. Rapidly fatal without treatment.
Erythema multiforme: An immunologically activated rash that appears as target lesions on the skin, sometimes accompanied by mucosal inflammation (Stevens-Johnson syndrome).
Kawasaki disease: See Kawasaki Disease p. 110.

P **Treatment for most viral exanthems is supportive, whereas treatment for bacterial infections almost always includes antibiotics.**
Aspirin is contraindicated to prevent Reye syndrome.

Admit pts with measles with pneumonia or encephalitis, or any suspected meningococcemia.

Obtain an echocardiogram and consult cardiology if you suspect rheumatic fever.
Lifetime penicillin prophylaxis will be required to prevent further GAS infections.

S **What symptoms is child having?**
Kawasaki disease (KD) has a constellation of symptoms that will help make the
diagnosis. The pt must have fever (>104°F) for 5 days and four of the following five
criteria:
- Bilateral nonpurulent conjunctivitis
- Oral lesions (oropharyngeal erythema, dry erythematous cracked fissured lips)
- Cervical lymphadenopathy (least common)
- Erythematous truncal rash
- Hand and feet changes (swelling of the digits and later periungual desquamation)

How old is child?
KD usually occurs between 6 months to 6 years. Never seen in children older than age 8.

O **Examine pt's general appearance and check vital signs.**
If pt is afebrile or not irritable, he or she is unlikely to have KD.

Perform a generalized PE, paying particular attention to the following areas:
Eyes: The bulbar conjunctiva should be erythematous and swollen but without
discharge.
Oral cavity: The lips are often red, swollen, and cracked. Oropharynx may be diffusely
erythematous, and there is often a strawberry tongue (red with stippling like a
strawberry).
Neck: Only 60% have the cervical lymphadenopathy, but when present it is usually
striking. It can be unilateral or bilateral, and a single lymph node should measure
>1.5 cm. It will likely be tender to palpation, but it should not be fluctuant because
this is a nonsuppurative adenopathy.
Skin: There is no specific rash in KD, so it is often referred to as a polymorphous rash.
It is usually erythematous and can resemble the rashes of measles (maculopapular),
scarlet fever (sandpaper-like), erythema multiforme (target-shaped lesions), etc.
Hand and feet changes: The palms and soles may be erythematous or indurated (hard to
the touch). They are often swollen, and desquamation (peeling) of the digits is often
seen, but usually in later stages of disease.

Look for these other PE signs:
Heart murmur: Associated with rare acute mitral insufficiency
Jaundice: Rare obstructive jaundice secondary to hydrops of the gallbladder or hepatitis

Check the labs. There are no diagnostic studies for KD, but the following are suggestive:
Thrombocytosis: Usually in the range of 600,000 to more than 1 million.
Elevated WBC: May be elevated to between 20,000 to 30,000. Erythrocyte
sedimentation rate and CRP may also be elevated.
Sterile pyuria: U/A shows WBCs without infection.
Aseptic meningitis (although not the kind commonly referred to when discussing a viral
or fungal etiology): If a lumbar puncture was performed, WBCs are often present,
again without infection. It is common although not frequently checked.

Kawasaki Disease
A medium-vessel vasculitis with characteristic symptoms as noted above. Etiology is
unknown, but many suspect an undiscovered infectious cause.

Avoidable Sequelae
Treatment is fairly benign, but the consequences of untreated disease can be life
  threatening.
This disease is often described in three stages:
  • *Acute stage:* Most of the above signs and symptoms associated with this stage.
  • *Subacute stage:* The fever, rash, and lymphadenopathy resolve and the vasculitis
    begins, causing coronary artery aneurysms (ectasias). This typically occurs
    between days 11 and 24 of the illness. Myocardial and endocardial inflammation
    can occur in 20% to 25% of pts. When these coronary artery aneurysms are
    associated with thrombocytosis, the pt is at risk for coronary artery obstruction
    and myocardial infarction.
  • *Late stage:* Coronary artery obstruction (myocardial infarction) occurs in this
    stage if the aneurysms do not resolve.
Treatment does not completely prevent aneurysms, but the risk is dramatically reduced.
Infants with KD (6 months to 1 year) might not display even four of five criteria
  (atypical KD) but should be treated anyway, because their risk of aneurysm is even
  higher.

Differential diagnosis of fever, rash, and conjunctivitis +/−
lymphadenopathy:

- Toxic shock syndrome	- Scarlet fever	- Rocky Mountain spotted fever
- Lyme disease	- Measles	- Erythema infectiosum
- Rubella	- Roseola	- Epstein-Barr virus
- Enterovirus	- Adenovirus	- Stevens-Johnson syndrome
- Serum sickness	- Systemic lupus	- Drug reaction
	erythematosus	

P **Admit and immediately begin treatment with intravenous
immunoglobulin (IVIG), 2 g/kg over 10 to 12 hrs qd and high-dose
aspirin, 20–25 mg/kg/dose qid.**
IVIG-only therapy has been shown to decrease the risk of coronary artery aneurysm.
Aspirin will provide both anti-inflammatory and antithrombotic effects.

Perform an echocardiogram.
If it is normal, the pt may have an appointment to repeat an echocardiogram in 6 to
  8 weeks.

After the child is afebrile 4 to 5 days, the aspirin dose can be decreased.
3 to 5 mg/kg once a day and can be discharged on this dose. This will continue the
  antithrombotic effects.
If the follow-up echocardiogram is negative for coronary lesions, the aspirin can be
  stopped. If coronary abnormalities are detected, the aspirin will be continued
  indefinitely. A pediatric cardiology specialist should determine the pt's treatment.

Remember that children on aspirin are at risk for Reye syndrome.
An autoimmune hepatitis with associated nonketotic hypoglycemia if they contract
  influenza or varicella. Instruct parents to call their pediatrician at the first sign of
  illness.

S **Which is first: the itch or the rash?**
Atopic dermatitis, a form of eczema, is sometimes called the itch that rashes, but this
   phenomenon could also occur in systemic disease such as liver, kidney, or endocrine
   disorders.

Does the itching prevent sleep?
Scabies, eczema, and urticaria can all be severe enough to awaken the pt from sleep.

Where is the rash?
Scabies spares the head and neck and occurs especially at the interdigital webs and
   other areas known as intertriginous zones:

- Penile shaft	- Wrists	- Elbows
- Groin	- Natal cleft	- Axillae

Atopic dermatitis occurs in the popliteal and antecubital fossae, around the eyes and
   ears, and in the various skin folds and creases.

When did the rash start?
Scabies is often chronic, with pruritus sometimes continuing for weeks after treatment.
Urticaria is often acute but can recur.
Atopic dermatitis tends to be chronic with a difficult-to-remember start date.

Does anyone else have the rash?
Scabies can occur in multiple family members, but often the first case in a family will
   precede the others by about a month, about the time it takes for someone to become
   sensitized to the infestation.

Does anyone in the family have allergic disease?
A strong family history of asthma, allergies, eczema, or other allergic problems is
   suspicious or at least supportive of the diagnosis of atopic dermatitis.

Are there any associated symptoms?
If pts are having any malaise, fatigue, weight loss, or other systemic symptoms, then
   consider illnesses such as cancer, autoimmune, liver, renal, and endocrine diseases.
If pts are having urticaria, angioedema, and symptoms of shortness of breath or
   impending doom, consider anaphylaxis and treat with urgency (see Anaphylaxis
   p. 60).

What medicines is the child taking?
Medication reaction is another thing to consider when pruritic rash exists.
Antibiotics such as penicillins, cephalosporins, and sulfa drugs are all common culprits.

O **Carefully examine the rash and note its distribution.**
Scabies: Look for burrows on the wrists, penis shaft, elbows, axillae, between fingers,
   feet, groin, perineum, and natal cleft.
Atopic dermatitis: Look for a dry, scaly rash in the folds and creases of the body, areas
   such as the antecubital fossae, popliteal fossae, and around the ears and eyes.
Urticaria and the other pruritic rashes do not seem to follow a particular distribution.

**Test for dermatographism by running the back of your pen on the pt's
arm with some pressure. If a wheal forms at the site within minutes,
the test is positive.**
Suggestive for urticaria/allergic rash

Consider the following lab tests:
BUN/Cr: Elevated BUN suggests uremia, which can cause itching.
Liver tests and hepatitis panel: An elevated bilirubin can cause itching.

A **All of these rashes can be diagnosed by exam:**

Scabies: Burrows in interdigital webs, at the wrists, penis shaft, elbows, feet, groin, perineum, natal cleft, and axillae

Atopic dermatitis: A dry, scaly rash in the fossae and folds of the body. One of the most common rashes in childhood, it occurs in up to 10% of children. It is often associated with asthma and allergic rhinitis.

Urticaria: Pruritic wheals that tend to rise up and resolve within hours, only to rise up at a different site. They usually resolve with antihistamines.

Molluscum contagiosum: Papules with umbilicated centers, which spread from place to place on the skin with scratching. They are viral in origin.

Miliaria rubra: Patches of erythema with small papulovesicles; a common heat rash.

Lichen planus: Flat-topped papules and hypertrophic plaques on wrists, low back, eyelids, shins, scalp, and the head of the penis.

Differential diagnosis

Secondary to systemic diseases such as cancer (especially cutaneous T-cell lymphomas), liver disease (cholestasis), chronic renal failure, drug reactions, polycythemia, insect bites, parathyroid dysfunction, psychogenic pruritus, and opiate withdrawal

P **Scabies: Apply permethrin cream to all of skin for 12 hrs; wash sheets and clothes in hot water.**

This should ensure death for all of the infecting organisms. It is highly contagious, so consider treating all family members.

Atopic dermatitis: Apply moisturizing creams several times a day and pat (do not rub) dry after bathing.

If this is ineffective, short courses of mild topical steroids should alleviate symptoms.

Urticaria: Give antihistamines and try to find the cause.

Viral is the most common cause, but it is more likely that the cause will never be found.

Molluscum contagiosum: Advise pt (parent) to avoid scratching because it will spread the lesions.

The lesions may be removed but often resolve spontaneously in a matter of months.

Miliaria rubra: Expose affected area and allow it to dry and cool.
Lichen planus: Treat with topical corticosteroids.
Drug allergy: If it is suspected, stop the medication and wait to see if the rash improves.

S **Is there a rash, joint pain, abdominal pain, and blood in the urine?**
If so, it is very likely you have diagnosed Henoch-Schönlein purpura (HSP). At the very least, you should have rash and joint pain or abdominal pain.

What does the rash look like?
The rash should look like purple, well-circumscribed bruises that do not blanche.

Which joints hurt?
Usually it is the knees or ankles and it is symmetric.

Ask the pt to describe the abdominal pain
Usually described as crampy or colicky.

Any vomiting or blood in the stool?
Vomiting with abdominal pain occurs occasionally. It can be confused with appendicitis.
Blood and mucus in the stool are both common.

Is there any blood in the urine or any foaming of the urine in the toilet bowel?
Asymptomatic hematuria and/or proteinuria are common.

Has the child had any colds recently?
Many children report a recent upper respiratory infection, suggesting that a viral infection may lead to an immune disruption that causes HSP.

O **Perform a careful PE.**
Perform a good general exam, looking specifically to eliminate things such as sepsis, idiopathic thrombocytopenic purpura (ITP), and lupus.

Does the rash look typical for HSP?
Purpuric (nonblanching, bruise-like lesions +/− palpable) on the lower extremities
Petechiae (nonblanching pinpoint red lesions) could suggest ITP or other platelet disorder.
Macular rashes or any blanching rashes should suggest alternative diagnoses.
Malar rash on the face suggests systemic lupus erythematosus (SLE).

Is there any focal abdominal tenderness?
Abdominal pain that localizes to a particular area (e.g., RLQ) suggests alternative diagnoses like appendicitis, especially if there is guarding or peritoneal signs (see Abdominal Pain p. 72).

Are there any signs of arthritis?
Although mild joint swelling may occur, warmth and redness suggest alternative diagnoses.

Check pertinent labs:
U/A: In HSP may see hematuria (either gross or microscopic) and/or proteinuria. If there is a suspicion of sepsis, send the urine for culture.
BUN and Cr to evaluate renal function
CBC, and if the suspicion is high enough for sepsis, also send a blood culture.
IgA is elevated in 50% of pts with HSP. May help confirm the diagnosis.
Anti ENA-4 panel (anti-dsDNA, anti-Smith, anti-Ro, and anti-La) and antinuclear antibody (ANA) if suspect SLE.
Skin biopsy showing leukocytoclastic vasculitis can confirm the diagnosis.
PT, PTT, antiphospholipid antibody to rule out other causes of easy bruising.

Henoch-Schönlein Purpura (HSP)

An IgA-mediated small-vessel vasculitis characterized by four classic findings:
- Purpuric rash on the lower extremities
- Symmetric arthralgia of the large joints of the lower extremities
- Crampy abdominal pain with vomiting
- Asymptomatic hematuria

Symptoms can vary, but at minimum, the rash is required for diagnosis.
A biopsy of the skin should show a leukocytoclastic vasculitis.

Differential diagnosis

Several alternative diagnoses have already been mentioned. Of these, the most important to rule out either by H&P or with labs and further studies is sepsis, especially meningococcal.

Other diagnoses to consider are:
- ITP: Petechiae, mucosal bleeding, thrombocytopenia

- SLE: A good mnemonic is MD NO PARISH ANA ("Dr., don't let ANA die"):
  - *M*alar rash
  - *D*iscoid rash
  - *N*euro (like seizures, psychosis)
  - *O*ral ulcers
  - *P*hotophobia
  - *A*rthritis
  - *R*enal (like proteinuria)
  - *I*mmune (like false + VDRL, anti-dsDNA)
  - *S*erositis (pleuritis, pericarditis)
  - *H*eme (like thrombocytopenia, leukopenia)
  - *ANA* +

- Other vasculitic processes, such as Goodpasture disease or Wegener granulomatosis, may lead to hematuria, abdominal pain, or other nonspecific complaints.
- *Juvenile rheumatoid arthritis:* See Limping in Child without History of Trauma p. 116.
- *Appendicitis:* RLQ abdominal pain with peritoneal signs, vomiting, and fever
- *Tuberculosis:* Fever, night sweats (enough to need to change the bedsheets), chronic nonproductive cough, hemoptysis, and weight loss
- *Mesenteric:* Can cause crampy abdominal pain.
- *TTP/HUS:* Microangiopathic hemolytic anemia, renal failure, +/− mental status changes
- *Leukemia:* Can present with many of the same symptoms as HSP, so checking a CBC is a good idea for many reasons. CBC may show blasts.
- *Child abuse:* Can also cause many of the same symptoms of abdominal pain, lower extremity bruising, hematuria, and joint pain (see Physical Abuse p. 122).

P   **Observe without treatment.**

After the diagnosis is made, the child is followed for possible loss of renal function and to rule out more dangerous things on the differential diagnosis, but usually the symptoms resolve without incident.

May start prednisone 1 mg/kg/day if the pt needs symptomatic relief.

The worst outcome is usually related to worsening of renal function, even to the point of renal failure. In these cases, there is no proven treatment but prednisone, cyclosporin, and even renal transplant. All have been tried, but there is no consensus regarding proper treatment.

S **What bit/stung the child?**

Insects that sting: Bees, wasps, hornets, yellow jackets, ants

Insects that bite: Mosquitoes, fleas, lice

Arachnids that sting: Scorpions, ticks

Arachnids that bite (spiders): Black widow, brown recluse

Venomous snakes: Rattlesnakes, cottonmouth, copperhead, diamondback

Nonvenomous snakes: Garter snake, gopher snake, king snake

Mammals: Human; bat; rat; cat; dog

Where was the child when bite or sting occurred?

- Grassy area with shrubs: ticks   - Ocean or beach: jellyfish or stingray
- In dark areas or in or near firewood piles: spiders or scorpions

How old is the child?

The same amount of venom that may only cause minor symptoms in an adult could kill a small child.

Does the pt have any other problems or complaints?

Fever is a concerning symptom suggesting superinfection of the bite.

Anaphylaxis (see p. 60): Should be addressed emergently if suspected.

Spider bites: Pain, swelling, paresthesias, headache, nausea, abdominal rigidity

Snake bites: Severe swelling can cause compartment syndrome. See Limb Trauma p. 120.

Stingray/jellyfish stings: Nausea/vomiting, syncope, paralysis, muscle cramps, seizure

Scorpion stings: Nystagmus, mydriasis (blurred vision), hypersalivation, dysphagia, diaphragmatic paralysis (trouble breathing), restlessness, seizure

 Perform a general PE.

Inspect all areas carefully, especially areas with hair, for foreign bodies such as ticks or stingers.

Inspect skin for rashes, bites, or breaks.

- *Tick bites:* Look carefully for the tick, because it may still be there.
- *Cat or snake bites:* Are puncture wounds (high risk for infection).
- *Spider bites:* Often cause visible small breaks in the skin with central pallor.
- *Stingray stings:* May be pale, red, or blue, and swollen with local lymphadenopathy.
- *Jellyfish stings:* cause a red, raised, pruritic, painful rash.
- *Insect stings:* Look for a stinger and local angioedema.
- *Scorpion stings:* Cause a purpuric plaque, which progresses to ulceration and necrosis (the amount of venom is represented by the diameter of the lesion) with lymphatic streaking.
- If the child has been in a fight, look at the fingers and hands and ears for closed-fist, finger tendon, and ear cartilage injuries.

With breaks in the skin, look specifically for signs of infection such as redness, streaking, warmth, or swelling around the wound. Look for pus or discharge from the wound.

X-ray the area of injury, looking for embedded foreign bodies or broken bones.

Check labs: With envenomations for signs of infection or hemolysis (CBC), electrolyte abnormalities (lytes), hypoglycemia (glucose), rhabdomyolysis (CK), renal failure (Cr), and bleeding diathesis and or hepatic injury (liver enzymes, PT, PTT).

ECG (if arrhythmia) and echocardiogram (if heart failure) with severe envenomations

A Animal-induced injury with or without envenomation. Avoidable sequelae include:

Ticks: Tularemia, babesiosis, ehrlichiosis, Lyme disease, tick paralysis, Colorado tick fever, Q fever, relapsing fever, Rocky Mountain spotted fever

Mosquitoes: Equine encephalitis, dengue fever, yellow fever, malaria

Stings or venoms: Anaphylaxis or systemic toxicity of the venom

Human bites: Closed-fist injuries can lead to septic joints, disabling damage to tendons.

Animal bites: Dog bites are high risk because they cause crushing injury. Consider treatment for rabies, especially with bats, skunks, raccoons, foxes, or any wild carnivore. Domesticated animals are less likely to cause rabies. With any dirty, open wound, consider tetanus (See Limb Trauma p. 121).

P Remove all ticks and stingers.

Grab as close to the skin as possible. Pull out slowly with forceps, and then clean the site thoroughly.

Soak stingray injuries in tolerably hot water to reduce pain.
Wash jellyfish stings in normal saline or acetic acid to inactivate stingers.

Plain water will release more toxin.

For human or animal bites, use lidocaine to numb the wound and clean thoroughly.

Irrigate with copious amounts of clean water and debride the wound.

Leave the wound open (unsutured), unless it is on the face.

Consult a hand surgeon if the injury occurred to the hand.

If suspicion is high enough, such as unprovoked wild animal attack, vaccinate.

Rabies is required for bats, rodents, and animals foaming at the mouth (dogs in the United States are unlikely to carry rabies).

Evaluate need for tetanus vaccination or immune globulin. See Limb Trauma p. 120.

Give Augmentin for 3 to 7 days with high-risk bites. Reevaluate in 24 to 48 hrs.

High risk: Punctures, wounds with redness/warmth, wounds in immunosuppressed pts

Give instructions to return sooner if signs of infection are noticed.
If swelling is occurring around the wound, elevate and decrease use of the affected limb and remove constricting clothing or jewelry.
If extensive necrosis or compartment syndrome occurs, consult a surgeon.

This will be most common with venomous stings and bites.

Rule out or treat anaphylaxis.

Hymenoptera venom is a common cause. See Anaphylaxis p. 60.

Give antivenin if snake, spider, or scorpion type can be identified and is available. Contraindicated treatments include cutting and attempting to suction venom, and using ice, alcohol, or tourniquets.

If rhabdomyolysis (spider bites) occurs, hydrate heavily with normal saline IV. If that fails then consult renal for dialysis.

Treat pruritus with antihistamines.

How old is the child?

This changes your differential somewhat. Toddlers and children will usually have an infection, whereas adolescents will usually have slipped capital femoral epiphysis (SCFE), Osgood-Schlatter, or a rheumatologic disorder like juvenile rheumatoid arthritis (JRA).

Where is the pain?

The location of the pain can give you an idea about where the pathology is, and this can help with the differential diagnosis. Keep in mind that knee pain can be referred hip pain and vice versa. If the child has either hip or knee pain, perform a good PE to discern the actual source of the pain. If the pain is not over a joint but instead over a long bone, consider osteomyelitis, fracture, or even cancer.

Is there any fever?

The presence of fever in a child with a limp helps promote diagnoses such as septic joint, osteomyelitis, and JRA.

The absence of fever suggests diagnoses such as SCFE, Osgood-Schlatter, and Legg-Calve-Perthes disease.

Has the child received steroids recently?

This increases the risk of avascular necrosis of the hip.

Perform a good PE.

After reviewing the vital signs and performing a good general PE, look specifically and carefully at the musculoskeletal exam for any signs of:

- *Septic joint:* Pain, swelling, warmth, redness, and decreased range of motion (ROM) over a single joint
- *Osteomyelitis:* Pain, swelling, warmth, and redness over an area of skin overlying a bone
- *JRA:* Swelling, warmth in any or several joints, lymphadenopathy, hepatosplenomegaly
- *SCFE:* Pain on internal rotation
- *Legg-Calve-Perthes:* Pain (in hip or knee) with weakness and decreased ROM in the hip
- *Osgood-Schlatter's:* Pain and localized swelling at the tibial tuberosity

Order the appropriate labs and studies:

Get an X-ray series (X-ray of *two or more* views, usually anteroposterior [AP] and lateral) of the joint.

SCFE: Get an AP and frog-leg view of the pelvis, looking for an "ice cream sliding off the cone" appearance to the epiphysis of the greater trochanter.

Legg-Calve-Perthes disease: Take an x-ray or MRI of the affected hip, looking for disruption, or worse, destruction of the femoral head.

To help differentiate septic joint, JRA, and osteomyelitis obtain a CBC with diff, CRP, blood culture, ESR, ANA, and rheumatoid factor (RF).

If the joint has palpable fluid, aspirate it and send for cell count and culture.

Osgood-Schlatter's: No imaging is necessary if classic findings present on exam.

Evaluate the cause of limping.

Septic joint: Fever with a single joint swollen, hot, and red. Elevated WBC, CRP, and ESR with a predominance of neutrophils and possibly bands on the peripheral smear. Blood culture and aspirate culture may or may not be positive. Joint aspirate should have >50,000 polymorphonuclear neutrophil leukocytes.

Osteomyelitis: Disruption of the cortex of the bone on x-ray with overlying erythema and fever. Blood cultures will likely be positive. Gram-positive organisms are most likely.

JRA: Note there are three types:

- Pauciarticular: <4 joints. If ANA is positive, there is increased risk of uveitis.
- Polyarticular: >4 joints. Similar to early rheumatoid arthritis, especially if RF is positive
- Systemic (Still's disease): More systemic with less joint complaints
- Mnemonic: WAFFL ME CHARMS.

- Weight loss	- Anemia	- Fatigue
- Fever	- Lymphadenopathy/leukocytosis	
- Myalgias	- ↑ESR	
- ↑CRP	- Hepatosplenomegal	- Anemia
- Rash	- Morning stiffness	- Serositis

SCFE: Hip or knee pain with decreased ROM and pain on internal rotation at the hip with classic x-ray findings. Very often associated with obesity.

Legg-Calve-Perthes: Pain in the hip or knee with disruption or destruction of the ball of the ball-and-socket joint of the hip. Most common in the 3- to 4-yr-old age group.

Osgood-Schlatter's: Tender nodule at the tibial tuberosity and knee pain, worse with running.

Differential diagnosis

Fracture: Although there is no history of it, trauma still may have occurred and either the child is not telling the parent, the parent is not telling the clinician, or it seemed insignificant.

Cancer: Consider bone tumor if there is a localized swelling or mass in the leg, and the x-rays show a cyst, mass invading the bone, or other suspicious lesion. Consider lymphoma or leukemia if the pt has other masses, hepatosplenomegaly, lymphadenopathy, or blasts on the peripheral smear. In the latter cases, pain comes from rapid bone marrow expansion.

P

Consult Orthopedics emergently for suspected septic joint.

Surgical treatment is required to save the joint. Do not wait to start antibiotics.

- Septic joints can easily progress to sepsis, especially in younger children.

Start cefazolin if osteomyelitis is suspected.

Chronic therapy and removal of infected orthopedic hardware will be required.

If JRA is suspected, call pediatric rheumatology for further workup and treatment.

Rule out cancer and infection before starting steroids.

For SCFE and Legg-Calve-Perthes, refer to Orthopedics for surgical intervention.

No weight bearing until after surgery.

Treat Osgood-Schlatter's with NSAID therapy.

This should effectively decrease the inflammation of the tibial tuberosity.

Reduce and cast all fractures and refer to Orthopedics for those fractures that may require surgery.

Refer to Child Protective Services if abuse is suspected (see Suspected Physical Abuse p. 122).

Refer all suspected malignancies to Oncology.

S **How did the head trauma occur?**

Mechanism of injury is important in judging expected severity (fall from couch vs. 3rd floor).

Consider child abuse if a story sounds strange, changes, or is inconsistent with the injury.

Did the pt lose consciousness?

Loss of consciousness (LOC) suggests significant injury. Talk to someone who witnessed the event. Ask if the child cried immediately or if he or she seemed awake the entire time.

If there were no witnesses and the pt is old enough to answer questions, ask what he or she remembers about the incident. Amnesia to any part of the event suggests LOC.

Did the pt have any posttraumatic events, such as a seizure or vomiting?

Contact seizures: Seizures that occur within seconds of the injury. They are benign.

Early posttraumatic seizures: Seizures that begin >1 minute after the trauma are clinically significant. Observe pt for risk of further seizures.

Vomiting: Short-term vomiting is also benign. Vomiting that persists for more than 4 hrs after the event is concerning.

Other posttraumatic events include:
- Headache (probably most common)   - Dizziness
- Cerebrospinal fluid leakage from the ears or nose (likely indicates a basilar skull fracture)
- Waning LOC

O **Evaluate pt's level of consciousness.**

This is probably the most important part of the PE in this pt. If pt is a well-appearing conscious child or adolescent brought in by a concerned parent, there is probably not much to worry about. However, if pt displays altered LOC even if Glasgow Coma Scale (GCS) is 15 (normal), careful observation and often interventions must be taken.

The GCS will help you assess pt (Table 8).

The maximum score is 15, the minimum is 3.

If pt has a GCS of 8 or less, the pt is unlikely to be able to protect own airway and should be intubated.

Look at vital signs.

Cushing's triad: A late sign of increased intracranial pressure (ICP) with bradycardia, hypertension, and abnormal respirations

Examine head for signs of trauma:

Hematoma: Feels like a hard, ovoid mass. It should be tender to palpation.

Step-off: Might indicate a depressed skull fracture.

Laceration: May need to be sutured or skin-clipped.

Fundoscopic exam: Look for sharp optic disc margins. Blurred margins suggest increased ICP. Retinal hemorrhages suggest shaken baby syndrome.

Ears: Hemotympanum (blood behind the tympanic membrane [TM]) or a ruptured TM with clear liquid discharge are both consistent with a basilar skull fracture.

Battle sign: An ecchymotic line (bruise) behind the ear that usually appears several hours after the trauma. It also suggests basilar skull fracture.

Raccoon eyes: Periorbital ecchymoses that also suggest basilar skull fracture.

Septal hematoma: A surgical emergency. Look in the nose for a bulging dark red or black septum.

Perform a complete neurologic exam, provided pt is conscious

Note any focal neurologic findings. Mnemonic is C MR CGR ("See Mr. Cougar"):
- Cranial nerves   - Motor   - Reflexes
- Cerebellar   - Gait   - Rhomberg   - Sensory

Although it is still controversial, all pts should get a head CT except:

Pts with a GCS of 15 who are not acting strangely, who did not lose consciousness at the scene, have a normal neurologic exam, no signs of basilar skull fracture on exam, no further vomiting, and no more than a mild headache or dizziness.

Table 8 Glasgow Coma Scale		
Eyes Open	**Motor**	**Verbal**
4 = Spontaneously	6 = Obeys Commands	5 = Oriented
3 = To Speech	5 = Localizes to Pain	4 = Confused
2 = To Pain	4 = Withdraws from Pain	3 = Words
1 = Closed	3 = (Decorticate) Flexor Posturing	2 = Sounds
	2 = (Decerebrate) Extensor Posturing	1 = Nonverbal
	1 = No Movement	

Blunt head trauma

Concussion: A normal head CT with mild persistent symptoms, headache, dizziness, etc.
Contusion: Found on head CT as a point of edema with or without bleed.
Epidural hematoma: Caused by a ruptured intracranial artery, usually the middle meningeal artery. Clinically characterized by an initial LOC, followed by a lucid interval, followed by waning consciousness. It shows up as a lentiform-shaped bleed on the head CT, compressing the brain. There may be midline shift of the brain.
Subdural hematoma: Caused by torn bridging veins between the brain and the dura. Characterized by a unilateral crescent-shaped bleed on CT scan, exerting minimal pressure on the brain.
Skull fracture, basilar, depressed, or nondepressed: Basilar skull fractures have a 10% risk of meningitis. Depressed skull fractures have an increased risk of seizures.

All of the above diagnoses, with the exception of concussion, require a neurosurgical evaluation. Pts with concussions may be sent home.

Parents should be given instructions to return if their child's consciousness wanes or changes, if the vomiting returns, or if the child has diplopia or ataxia.
Athletes who participate in contact sports should have a mandatory week off from activity. Two concussions within 1 week puts them at risk for sudden death.

Admit to a monitored bed all pts with:

GCS < 15, early posttraumatic seizure, skull fractures, all bleeds, persistent vomiting, dizziness, or abnormal neurologic exam

S **What was the mechanism of the injury?**
This will tell you how the accident happened, what limb was involved, etc.
The story will also be important in ruling out child abuse.

Can the child move the limb? If the leg is involved, can the child bear weight?
The ability to move or bear weight may give some indication about the severity of the injury.

O **Begin with a rapid but thorough general PE.**
It is important not to miss other possible sites of trauma. These could indicate that the injuries are more extensive than previously thought or that there is a pattern of the injuries that could be consistent with abuse.

Examine the affected limb.
The limb may be swollen, red, and warm at the site of trauma. It will almost certainly be tender. Point tenderness may indicate a fracture.
Skin breakage or obvious deformity might indicate a compound fracture.
Check to see if the limb has passive mobility and if the child will let you move it.
Nursemaid's elbow: Subluxed radial head caused by a traction injury on the arm of a toddler. The child will be holding the arm extended and internally rotated and will refuse to move it. X-rays are unnecessary unless you suspect a fracture. To reduce, hold the radial head, rapidly supinate and then flex the forearm; if that does not work, try pronation and then flexion. A click or pop is usually heard with successful reduction. It may take a few minutes for the child to start using the arm.
Perform a neurovascular examination distal to the site of injury. Check that pulses are equal to the contralateral side. Digits should be warm with brisk capillary refill after pressure, actively mobile by the pt, with no pain on passive movement, and have sensation.

Look carefully for broken skin.
If the skin is broken, look carefully for both fracture and foreign body.
Skin breakage puts the pt at risk for infection, including cellulitis and osteomyelitis.

Obtain x-rays of the affected limb in multiple views.
Order at least two views (AP and lateral usually called a "series," e.g., "Right hand series") of the affected area. Fractures and dislocations are not always seen on a single view.
In a toddler or infant with lower extremity trauma in which the site of injury is not obvious on PE, the entire lower extremity must be imaged.
If child indicates knee or hip pain, x-ray both joints. Pain can refer from one joint to the other.

A **Limb trauma. Assess for fracture.**
Traumas with no point tenderness and negative x-rays and intact neurovascular exams are likely to be sprains or ligamentous injuries.

Fracture type
Fractures can be:

- Transverse (perpendicular to   - Torus (buckling of the bone)
  the bone's length)   - Spiral (twisting injury)
- Longitudinal (parallel   - Oblique (diagonal)
  to the bone's length)
- Compound (fracture associated
  with a break in the skin)

The next three fractures only occur in pediatrics.
- *Greenstick:* Bone bends, leaving cortical disruption on only one side.
- *Bending:* Bone looks slightly more curved than it should.
- *Salter Harris (SH):* Fractures of the growth plate

There are five types of SH fractures. A good mnemonic is **SALTER**. For the mnemonic to work, think of the femur at the knee where "above" means toward the side of the growth plate with the metaphysis (the long part) and "below" means toward the short end of the bone.

- Type I: (*S*ame) no change in appearance of growth plate.
- Type II: (*A*bove) fracture occurs Above the growth plate (most common, ~70%).
- Type III: (*L*ow) fracture occurs beLow the growth plate.
- Type IV: (*T*hrough) fracture goes Through the growth plate (both above and below).
- Type V: (*E*mergency *R*oom or *R*ammed) fracture obliterates space of growth plate.

Evaluate for possible compartment syndrome or significant neurovascular injury.

Compartment syndrome: The swelling in one or more of the soft tissue compartments in the limb (spaces between facial planes) causes compression of the nerves and blood vessels in the compartment, leading to neurovascular damage. Pain on passive movement of the digits (most sensitive and specific), pallor, paresthesia, and absent or weak pulses all suggest the diagnosis.

- 4P's is a good mnemonic: Pain (with passive movement of digits), Paresthesia, Pallor, Pulselessness

Consult Orthopedics emergently for a fasciotomy if you suspect compartment syndrome.

P **Consult Orthopedics emergently for suspected compartment syndrome or neurovascular injury.**
Waiting may cost the pt a limb.

Cast simple fractures and provide Orthopedic follow-up.
For complex fractures (like open fractures), involve Orthopedics on a nonemergent basis.
Without orthopedic intervention, SH fractures have increased risk of poor growth because of the damage to the growth plate.

Recommend home treatment with Rest, Ice, Compression, and Elevation (RICE) and an NSAID like ibuprofen for all sprains or ligamentous injuries.
Suspected child abuse should be reported to the appropriate authorities.
See Suspected Physical Abuse p. 122.
Check the vaccination card and give tetanus prophylaxis if necessary (Table 9).
If the pt received all childhood vaccinations and has had the last one within the last 5 years, then they need nothing. If they have a small, contaminated wound and parents do not know the vaccination history, then the American Academy of Pediatrics recommends both Td and TIG be given.

Table 9 Vaccinations				
DtaP	**Small Clean Wounds**		**Contaminated or Large Wounds**	
Series	**Td**	**TIG**	**Td**	**TIG**
? or <3	Yes	No	Yes	Yes
≥3	No if in Last 10 yr	No	No if in Last 5 yr	No

S **Did the parents seek medical care in a timely fashion?**
One of your first clues to abuse is a delay in seeking care for a serious injury.

Does the story match the injury?
Think about whether the injury sustained is possible by the mechanism proposed.

Is the story inconsistent or vague in some way?
Another red flag for child abuse is different versions of the story from different people, or worse, different versions of the story from the same person. If the parents have no idea how this happened, that is also cause for suspicion or at least further investigation.

Is the child developmentally capable of the injury?
The child cannot have climbed up the stairs if he or she is not even rolling over yet.

Interview the child alone.
If children are old enough to tell the story themselves, they should be allowed to do so.

Who has access to the child?
It does not necessarily have to be the person who brought the child to the hospital who is at fault. There could be an aunt, uncle, cousin, friend, stepparent, or parent's significant other who was the abuser.

O **Carefully observe the interactions of the child and parent.**
If the parent does not show appropriate concern for the degree of the injury or exhibits inappropriate, angry, or abusive behavior with the child or siblings, that should be noted.

Examine the child carefully for signs of abuse.
Look for bruises in patterns caused by hands, hangers, extension cords, belt buckles, and so on.
Look for areas of local tenderness and or swelling over bones suggesting fractures, especially ribs, head, and extremities.
Bruises at different stages of healing or in atypical locations such as face, ears, upper arms, hands, thighs, feet, chest, abdomen, back

Look for other skin lesions.
Burns from immersion in hot water or brandings from hot objects such as the following are all injuries to be further investigated: irons, lighters, cigarette butts.
Also look for abrasions or bruising from gags, tourniquets, and other restraints.
Look carefully at the inside of the mouth/palate, anus, and genitalia for other signs of abuse (see Considering Sexual Abuse p. 124).

Obtain a skeletal series looking for fractures.
If you suspect abuse, it is often prudent, in younger children, to obtain a skeletal survey on which you may find multiple ages of fractures.

Consider head and abdominal CT.
If the pt has altered mental status, any focal neurologic deficit, or is an infant, obtain a head CT emergently to rule out an intracranial hemorrhage.
If there is any abdominal bruising or tenderness, consider an abdominal CT to rule out splenic, hepatic, duodenal, or other intra-abdominal injury.

Check pertinent labs.
With significant soft tissue injury, check a CK and Chem 7 to rule out rhabdomyolysis. With abdominal trauma, check an amylase and a lipase to rule out traumatic pancreatitis.

If pt is an infant, obtain an emergent ophthalmologic exam.
Infants are at risk for retinal hemorrhages if they are shaken. This is diagnostic of abuse.

A
Consider parental and child risk factors for abuse:
Parental risk factors: Drug use, alcoholism, history of being abused, poverty, psychosis, prior abuse

Risk factors for children: <3 yrs, chronic illness, not the abuser's birth child, congenital anomaly

Assess for signs of abuse on x-ray.
Many fractures can be consistent with abuse, but what you have to decide is whether the history matches the degree of injury.

Two patterns of fracture that are nearly always indicative of abuse:
- Multiple, unexplained fractures in a symmetric pattern in various stages of healing in the ribs and long bones.
- Bucket handle fractures: Metaphyseal chips are seen on the lateral and medial aspect of the long bone. This fracture is usually caused by violent shaking of the extremity.

Fractures that are highly suspicious include:
- Transverse or oblique fractures of the humerus or femur without a good story
- Rib fractures in children less than 5 yrs old. These are highly suspicious because they are rarely present even after falls or car accidents.

Differential diagnosis
Accidental trauma: Sometimes the child actually did trip and fall.

Mongolian spots: Nontender flat blue nevi that the pt has had since birth.

Ricketts and osteogenesis imperfecta: Lead to fragile bones/multiple fractures of different ages.

Bleeding diatheses (e.g., hemophilia): May have very significant bruises from minor trauma.

Cultural practices: Cupping and coining are examples of practices from other countries in which objects are heated and rubbed on the skin. The marks they leave may appear severe, but because they are performed with the intention to heal, they are not considered abuse.

P
Decide if you suspect child abuse.
You are obligated to report the suspected abuser to the appropriate state government agencies as well as to law enforcement. The pt should be admitted to the hospital for protection. Suspicion of abuse is enough to warrant a report. Abuse usually recurs and escalates with each episode, so next time the pt may not survive to make it to the hospital.

Carefully document the H&P and PE.
Write down direct quotes without grammatical corrections. Have the pt point to any body part named and describe where pt points. If pictures would be useful, take them. Be sure to include a picture of the face and to time and date the photograph.

S **Who is the reporting party and how was the abuse discovered?**
It is important to note whether the pt has told a parent about sexual abuse, versus the parent having suspicions aroused by physical evidence, or by the presence of another child being abused in the home. A child who is directly admitting abuse is likely to be telling the truth. If a child is going to lie, she or he will more often deny abuse.

Have you noted any behavioral changes in the child?
Young children may:

| - Have a recurrence of bedwetting | - Lose bowel/ bladder control | - Become irritable |
| - Become clingy | - Develop new feeding difficulties | |

With older children, one might see:

- Drop in grades	- Loss of concentration	- Worsening peer relationships
- Depression	- Suicidal ideation	- Inappropriate sexual behavior
- Substance abuse		

Has the parent found any suspicious physical evidence?
Often the parent will note discharge or blood in the daughter's underwear as a major physical sign. Other signs include:

| - New recurrent abdominal pain | - Dysuria | - Genital bruising |
| - Lesions (verrucous, ulcerative, etc.) | - Swelling | - Discharge |

Find out the details of the alleged abuse, including who is accused, when and where did it happen, have there been multiple episodes, and, if so, for how long it has been going on.
It is worth noting that as much as 80% of all child abuse is perpetrated by someone the child knows, and often someone they are close to, especially a family member.

Interview the pt.
A child who has been abused may feel extremely vulnerable. Some tips on interviewing include the following:

- Begin by establishing rapport. This may be done by discussing nonthreatening topics, playing with toys, or drawing pictures.
- Use the child's language when naming body parts.
- Proceed from general to specific questions. Make sure not to lead the child with your questions. Ask "and then what happened?" rather than "Did he touch your privates?"
- Do not interrupt if a child reports abuse, just let her or him talk. When the child is finished, ask about details of sexual contact including penetration and pain.
- Be supportive and reassuring.
- If the child has not disclosed, be supportive. Relate that you understand that some of the complaints may be secondary to sexual abuse. Discuss secrets, fears, and touching.

O **Perform a general PE before examining the genitalia**
Look for signs of physical abuse, including unusual bruises or bite marks.

It is important to note that for a full and appropriate genital exam, your hospital's specialist team should be called. If one is not available, look for the following:
Examine entire perineal region for lacerations, abrasions, bruising, or scarring. Pay particular attention to posterior vulvar fourchette, hymen, and anus.

Old injuries may have skin tags or scars.

Children heal extremely well, so absence of scars does not rule out a history of abuse.

A normal exam does not rule out abuse.

It is important again to note that this exam should, whenever possible, be done by a specialist, with a handheld magnifier, a light, a camera, and a colposcope.

Before and throughout the exam, tell the child exactly what you are going to do. Make sure she or he is okay with everything you are doing before you do it.

Send urine for U/A with microscopy, chlamydial/gonorrheal ligase chain reactions, bacterial culture, and, in females older than 8 years old, check a pregnancy test.

Microscopy may reveal sperm if there was recent vaginal penetration with ejaculation.

If any of the tests for sexually transmitted infections or pregnancy are positive, this is very helpful in court to prove the abuse occurred.

Check blood for rapid plasma reagin (serum test for syphilis) and HIV if the parent consents.

Although syphilis and HIV can be acquired congenitally, in this situation a positive test would be supportive of sexual abuse.

A **Suspected Sexual Abuse**

Sexual abuse is more common than usually thought. In their lifetimes, 1 in 3 women will suffer sexual abuse or rape. In males, the number is closer to 1 in 12. Perpetrators are usually male.

Differential diagnosis

Abuse must be ruled out before anything else. If you suspect abuse, it should be reported. Protecting the child from further abuse is the goal. To achieve this, it must be identified and proven. Although conditions such as Munchausen syndrome and Munchausen by proxy are possible, they are much less common and much less likely than abuse.

One scenario that can occur is the divorced parent accusing the other of sexually abusing the child. If the child denies the abuse and there are more physical findings, it is still nearly impossible to know whether the abuse is occurring or not, but in either case it should be reported and thoroughly documented.

P **After the exam, it is the medical professional's job to act as a counselor.**

It is critical that the child's interaction with the medical professional be as positive an experience as possible.

It is important to address abused children's guilt, fear, and shame. Explain that it is not their fault and that they are in a safe environment now. Refer the family to family therapy.

It can only be hoped that through therapy, the family will be able to heal these scars.

As far as reporting is concerned, state laws differ, but it can be assumed that your state makes the medical professional a mandatory reporter.

Your state will most likely require both telephone and written reporting to Child Protective Services and the police.

Document everything thoroughly (when possible, use direct quotes without grammatical corrections), and photographs are also extremely helpful to prove a case in court.

V

Pediatric Ward

S **Were there any problems yesterday?**

This is a good question for anyone who saw the pt the night before (e.g., parent, nurse, doctor).

Does the pt have any pain? Has the pain been well-controlled?

Assess whether the pt has pain, where it is, if it is well-controlled, and if it has changed.

When was the last bowel movement?

Constipation is a common avoidable problem in the hospital.

How is the pt eating? Is he or she hungry?

This is a soft indicator that there might be more problems. Sick people lose their appetites.

Does the pt have any concerns or questions?

Gives an idea of how much the pt knows and an opportunity to inform or reassure.

Ask pt and parent about the child's condition and why he or she is in the hospital.

Assesses the pt/parent's understanding so that you can explain more clearly if necessary. Maintaining good communication avoids problems and ultimately leads to more effective therapy.

O **Review the chart quickly.**

Look at the notes (by consulting services, cross-covering doctors, the Attending, etc.) that have been written since your last note so you will know about important changes or updates.

Look at the orders for any new orders since the last time you saw the chart. Find out why the changes were made. Be sure to know meds, what they are, and why your pt is on them.

Look at the nursing notes for any information that may not be in the doctor's notes.

Review the vital signs and ins and outs from the night before.

Note any abnormalities in the vital signs, investigate possible causes, and notify the resident.

Examine the pt carefully.

Keep in mind your initial exam of the pt and note any changes.

See Table 10 for abbreviations for the PE (see Abbreviations for more).

In general: 1+ is < average, 2+ is about average, and 3+ is > average.

Review the pt's laboratories and microbiology results.

Again, note any abnormalities and investigate possible causes.

Look at all of the x-rays and other studies done on the pt.

By seeing them yourself, you can better understand and relay the official report.

A **Diagnosis:** _____, **Hospital Day:** _____

Assess for improvement.

If pt is not getting better, then the treatment plan may need to be reassessed.

Assess reason for continued hospitalization.

If you do not have a good reason why pts are still in the hospital, then they should go home.

Know what needs to be done to get the pt home or out of the hospital.

An efficient workup or treatment can only occur if you have a clear plan.

Be sure to address all of the pt's or parents' concerns.

If the pt/parent is dissatisfied, usually you have missed something or they think you have. It is important to clear up the misunderstanding in either case.

Parents are often better able to observe changes in their children, so listen to them.

P **Address any problems, pain, abnormal vitals, PE findings, labs, micro results, or studies found while gathering data to write your note.**
Note problems or abnormalities, and investigate possible causes.

Gather all of your data and write your note.
Subjective: Things told to you by the pt, parents, nurses, or other doctors
Objective: Data such as vitals, ins and outs, PE, labs, micro, and studies
Assessment: Summarize diagnoses and whether they are improving, worsening, or static
Plan: Summarize what will be done for each of the problems the pt has
Record information such as medicines, IV fluids, diet, and hardware.
Organize the assessment and plan by problem list or by systems:
- Neuro = Neurologic
- Resp = Respiratory
- CV = Cardiovascular
- FEN/GI = Fluids Electrolytes Nutrition/Gastrointestinal
- Renal/GU = Renal/Genitourinary
- Heme/ID = Hematologic/Infectious Disease
Be sure to time, date, and sign your note.
The note should be a summary showing both what has and will happen.

Table 10 Abbreviation for the Physical Exam*		
VS = Vital Signs	**P** or **HR** = Pulse/Heart Rate	**T** = Temperature
BP = Blood Pressure	**R** or **RR** = Respiratory Rate	**PS** = Pain Score
Gen = General Appearance	**HEENT** = Head Eyes Ears Nose Throat	
TM = Tympanic Membrane	**NCAT** = Normocephalic Atraumatic	
OP = Oropharynx	**AFSFO** = Anterior Fontanelle Soft Flat and Open	
EOMi = Extraocular Muscles intact	**PERRLA** = Pupils Equal Round Reactive to Light and Accommodation	
CV = Cardiovascular	**RRR** = Regular Rate and Rhythm	
SM = Systolic Murmur	φ **M/R/G/C** = No Murmurs/Rubs/Gallops/Clicks	
B = Bilateral	**Lungs CTA** = Lungs Clear to Auscultation	
L = Left **R** = Right	+ **BS NT ND** = Positive Bowel Sounds Nontender Nondistended	
Abd = Abdomen	**NFEG/NMEG** = Normal Female/Male External Genitalia	
NRT = Normal Rectal Tone	**CVA** = Costovertebral Angle	
Ext = Extremities	φ **C/C/E** = No Cyanosis/Clubbing/Edema	
TTP = Tender to Palpation	**ROM** = Range of Movement **MAE** = Move All Extremities	
CN = Cranial Nerves	**DTR** = Deep Tendon Reflexes	

*Note: Exam headings are underlined.

S **When was the last time the child urinated? How many times in the last 24 hrs?**

If it has been more than 6 to 8 hrs since the child's last void, this is concerning and consistent with significant dehydration. Try to quantify how much less urine output (UOP) the pt has compared to normal.

Is the child making tears when he or she cries?

If the child is screaming and crying during the exam but not making a single tear, that will be another clue to the child's level of dehydration. Children less than 3 months of age may or may not produce tears making this an unreliable marker in this age group.

Is the child having vomiting, diarrhea? How many times per day? Is the child febrile?

If the child is having continued losses, then it is important to keep track of them and replace them so that you do not fall even further behind than you already are.

Fever represents an increase in the metabolic rate and diaphoresis, thus increasing the insensible losses.

Is the child eating and/or drinking?

If the child is eating and drinking, you may be able to orally replace the fluids being lost, but otherwise you may have to rehydrate intravenously.

Has the child lost weight, and do the parents remember a recent weight to compare with today's?

If you are fortunate enough to have a weight from 2 days ago that is 10% higher than today's weight, then it is easy to assess the degree of dehydration. It is 10%. For example, if a child weighed 12 kg 2 days ago and now weighs 10.5 kg, then the degree of dehydration is 12.5%.

O **Do a focused PE to assess dehydration.**

Signs to look for on PE to assess dehydration include:

- Hypotension
  (often a late and ominous sign)
- Altered mental status
- No tears when crying
- Sunken anterior fontanelle
  (children < 18 months)

- Tachycardia
- Dry mucus membranes
- Poor skin turgor
- Poor capillary refill

Check U/A, looking specifically for urine specific gravity (SG).

The more concentrated the urine (SG > 1.020), the more dehydrated the child is likely to be.

Check serum electrolytes, BUN, and creatinine.

Examine the lytes and replace any potassium or other electrolyte deficits. If there is hypernatremia, you can also calculate a **free water deficit = pt's wt × % dehydration**. The BUN/Cr ratio can also be a clue suggesting dehydration if the ratio of those two is greater than 10.

Examine for the cause of dehydration. It is often obvious (diarrhea, vomiting, or refusal to take any oral intake).

A   Assess degree of dehydration (Table 11).

Table 11 Degrees of Dehydration			
Dehydration	**%**	**Signs/Symptoms**	**Urine Specific Gravity**
Mild	5%	Dry mucus membranes, ↓UOP	1.020–1.030
Moderate	5–10%	Tachycardia, sunken fontanelle and eyes	>1.030
Severe	>10%	AMS, orthostatic, poor capillary refill	>1.035

P   Maintain your pt's daily fluid balance and rehydrate if necessary.

In reality, many dehydrated children can be orally rehydrated. But if the child is unable to tolerate oral fluids or if he or she is NPO for a procedure, then IV fluids are required.

Bolus if orthostatic or hypotensive

If severe dehydration exists, then bolus 20 cc/kg normal saline until orthostasis is corrected or the pt begins to urinate. After doing this three times for a total of 60 cc/kg, consider changing to colloid or blood for continued volume replacement. These boluses should not be added to the calculated fluid deficit.

Calculate fluid deficit using the three components of fluid replacement.

Initial deficit: Multiply the pt's weight by the assessed degree of hydration. So a 10-kg child who has severe dehydration has approximately a 1 kg = 1 L (remember that 1 L of water weighs 1 kg) deficit. This deficit should be replaced over 24 hrs, with the first half going in over the first 8 hrs and the second half going in over the next 16 hrs.

Maintenance fluids: 100 cc/kg/day or 4 cc/kg/hr for the first 10 kg, 50 cc/kg/day or 2 cc/kg/hr for the second 10 kg, and finally, 20 cc/kg/day or 1 cc/kg/hr for each remaining kg.

- Therefore, a 43-kg person should receive 1000 + 500 + 460 = 1960 cc per day.
- The same 43-kg person should receive an hourly maintenance of 40 + 20 + 23 = 83 cc/hr.
- 83 × 24 = 1992, so the numbers are fairly close.

Ongoing losses: Usually, if a pt is vomiting or stooling large amounts, keep track of the amount of the losses and replace them cc/cc with normal saline.

In summary, if a 21-kg child is 10% dehydrated, calculate the fluid replacement as:

- Deficit: 21 kg × 10% = 2.1 L, first half in first 8 hrs and second half in next 16 hrs
- Maintenance would be 40 + 20 + 1 = 61 cc/hr

So for the first 8 hrs, the rate would be 2100 cc/2 = 1050 cc/8 hrs = 131 + 61 = 192 cc/hr. Over the next 16 hrs, the rate should be 2100/2 = 1050/16 = 65.6 + 61 = 127 cc/hr with $D5\frac{1}{2}$ NS (with 20 mEq KCl/L added after the first void to ensure that the kidneys are working normally).

Total ongoing losses every 8 hours and give them back, cc for cc with normal saline over the next 2 to 4 hrs.

If the child is less than 4 months old, use $D5\frac{1}{4}$ NS as the fluid because the kidneys are not yet fully developed and less able to concentrate the urine.

An exception to this is any child of any age with hydrocephalus, ventriculoperitoneal shunt, or other neurosurgical pathology. In these children, given the increased risk of cerebral edema with hypotonic fluids, use only NS or D5NS for fluids regardless of the age.

S　**Does the pt have any pain? Rate the pain on a scale of 1 to 10.**
Assesses the severity of the pain so you can address and assess pain relief.

Ask the pt to point with one finger to where the pain hurts most.
Pain location will help immensely with the differential diagnosis.

Try to describe the pain: is it sharp, dull, crampy, or burning?
The description of the pain is useful when generating a diagnosis because certain
etiologies of pain have very different character. Dull chest pain has different
implications than sharp chest pain.

Does the pain travel anywhere?
Pain radiation can suggest neuropathic pain, such as pain radiating down the leg from
a pinched nerve in the spine, or it can suggest pancreatitis or dissecting aortic
aneurysm such as epigastric pain radiating to the back.

When did the pain start?
Abdominal pain for 5 years is less worrisome than abdominal pain for 1 to 2 days.

How long does each episode of pain last?
If pain lasts seconds, it is much less worrisome than hours.

How often do the pain episodes occur?
Pain occurring once a month versus once an hour is less worrisome.

Is the pain getting worse, better, or staying the same?
If the pain is getting worse, then you have less time to evaluate and treat it.

What is the pt usually doing when the pain starts?
The context or circumstances when the pain starts can be an important clue.

**Does anything make the pain worse or better? With activity, lying still,
or certain position?**
Exacerbating factors are helpful information for generating the differential diagnosis.

**Has the same pain ever happened before? If the pain occurred before,
what was done about it and what was it caused by? How is the pain
different this time?**
If this pain is similar to a previously diagnosed episode, that diagnosis may be the same
this time also, so it is worth knowing and considering.

O　**Perform a good general PE, but carefully examine the location of the
pain:**
Neck pain: Look for signs of meningitis or trauma and rule out both. Consider
checking a cervical spine film.
Extremity pain: Look carefully for masses, signs of infection (cellulitis), or signs of
trauma.
Joint pain: Examine for loss of function, range of motion, or weakness, as well as for
signs of arthritis.
Knee or hip pain: Examine both to assure that the knee pain is not actually referred hip
pain.
Abdominal pain: Examine for peritoneal signs (see Abdominal Pain p. 72).
Back pain: See if movement of the leg at the hip causes radiating pain to the toes,
suggesting neuropathic pain from a pinched nerve (unlikely in children without a
history of trauma).

A **Carefully investigate the possible causes of the pain and address them.**
Exclude the most dangerous possibilities such as peritonitis or appendicitis.

Differential diagnosis
Organic pain: Secondary to an organic cause, usually related to tissue damage.
Neuropathic pain: Results from neuronal injury, usually causes burning and/or
  hypersensitivity.
Malingering: The pt is simply making it up. Often associated with avoidance of an averse
  stimulus (e.g., school, juvenile hall, home if being abused) or for narcotic addiction.

P **Treat the pain.**
Even if the pain is dangerous (e.g., appendicitis) be sure to treat the pain during the
  workup.
Abbreviations:

- po = by mouth	- pr = per rectum	- IV = intravenous
- IM = intramuscular	- SQ = subcutaneous	- prn = as needed
- q = each	- qhs = at bedtime	- qd = once a day
- bid = 2 × a day	- tid = 3 × a day	- qid = 4 × a day

Mild Pain:
  • Acetaminophen: 10–15 mg/kg/dose (adult 650 mg) po/pr q4h prn
  • Ibuprofen: 10 mg/kg/dose (adult 200–800 mg) po q6h prn mild pain
Moderate Pain:
  • Ketorolac (Toradol): 0.4–1 mg/kg/dose (adult 15–30 mg) IV/IM q6h prn mod
    pain (max dose 40 mg/day, max duration 5 days, use only > age 2 yr old)
  • Naproxen: 2.5–10 mg/kg/dose (adult 500 mg po) q8-12h (max 1250 mg/day) prn
    mod pain (use only over the age of 2 yr old)
  • Acetaminophen with Codeine: 0.5–1 mg/kg/dose q4-6h (adult 2 tabs of the
    Tylenol #3 formulation) prn mod pain
Severe Pain:
  • Hydrocodone/Acetaminophen (Vicodin): 0.4–0.6 mg/kg/day divided tid or qid
    (adult, 2 tabs q4h) prn severe pain
  • Morphine: 0.05–0.1 mg/kg po/IM/SQ/IV q4h prn severe pain
  • Meperidine (Demerol): 1–1.5 mg/kg (max 150 mg) IM/SQ/PO q3-4h prn
If the pt weighs >40 kg, check that you are not giving more than the adult dose.
Patient-controlled analgesia should be used with severe pain whenever possible. It is a
  safe and effective way of controlling severe in-hospital pain.
Consider long-acting oral morphine or fentanyl (Duragesic) patches, before
  discharging a pt, if need to control chronic severe pain, as in cancer.

If you have chosen to give narcotic analgesics, always consider the side
effects.
If coma or a serious decrease in respiratory drive occurs, administer naloxone (Narcan)
  0.1 mg/kg/dose IV or IM. The half-life of Narcan is short, so you may need to repeat
  the dose.
Assume constipation will occur if the pt is using narcotics, and preventively start on a
  high-fiber diet and or docusate or other anticonstipation regimen. If it still occurs,
  treat with milk of magnesia or magnesium citrate.

S **What type of appendicitis did pt have?**

The type of appendicitis determines the postoperative course and management:

- *Acute appendicitis:* An infected appendix that has not yet perforated
- *Perforated appendicitis:* Appendix ruptures, releasing pus into abdomen
- *Gangrenous appendicitis:* A necrotic appendix, treated as a perforated appendicitis postop

Ask the pt to rate his or her level of pain.

Narcotics are usually required. Assess pain control frequently postop.

Acute appys tend to have less pain (due to less preop inflammation) than perf'd appys.

Has the pt passed gas or had a bowel movement yet?

Passing gas (flatus) or stool indicates gut motility, a sign of recovery. Acute appys tend to experience increasing motility within 48 hours postop. Perf'd appys may take longer.

Is the pt hungry? Does the pt think he or she can eat, or does he or she still feel nauseated?

Post-op ileus: When the bowel is manipulated during surgery, it causes a period of immotility during which the pt will not be hungry and may have nausea and vomiting.

Small bowel obstruction: Presents postop as frequent bilious (green) emesis and a distended abdomen. Obtain a KUB, place a nasogastric tube to suction, and get an emergent surgical consult. This is more common in pts with perf'd appys.

Recovery: When the pt begins to have flatus and regains appetite, he or she can be advanced meal by meal from ice chips to clear liquid to a regular diet.

Is the pt ambulating?

Walking should be encouraged. If the pt is not walking around by postop day 2, there is a risk for complications such as atelectasis and deep vein thrombosis (DVT).

O **Check for fever.**

In a postop acute appy, fever most likely indicates ongoing infection.

- Pts with perf'd appys can be expected to spike fevers for several days as their bodies deal with the contaminated peritoneal space caused by the rupture of the appendix.

Also consider the postsurgical causes of fever mnemonic, Five W's:

- *W*ind (atelectasis)	- *W*ater (UTI)	- *W*ound (wound
- *W*onder drugs (drug fever)	- *W*alking (DVT)	infection)

With that in mind, get the appropriate workup: chest x-ray, urine, blood, and wound cultures.

If fever is not present, assure that the pt is not tachycardic.

If pain control is good, then tachycardia is concerning for intravascular volume depletion, which is common in perf'd appys due third spacing. If it occurs, be sure to replace the volume.

Perform a PE, with a focus on the pt's lungs, abdomen, and extremities.

Lung exam: Should have equal breath sounds bilaterally, with good air entry without rales, rhonchi, or decreased breath sounds. If the lung exam is abnormal, check O_2 sat and chest x-ray.

Abdominal exam: Perform gently, check carefully for distention (may be associated with scrotal or labial edema). Examine wound site for dehiscence, erythema, or drainage.
Extremities exam: Examine for edema or abnormal capillary refill time (>2 seconds).

Check the labs.

Acute appys might only require one day of labs postop to make sure the WBC count decreased appropriately, representing resolution of the infection.
Perf'd appys require the following labs daily:
- Chem 7: Will give you information about this pt's fluid status. Hyponatremia with an elevated BUN is consistent with a pt who has third-spacing fluid.
- CBC: Persistently elevated WBC count represents ongoing infection and often correlates with continued fevers.

A **Acute or Perforated appendicitis, postop day** _____
Ensure that you assess the four following areas:
- *Pain:* Well-controlled?
- *Fever:* Ongoing infection versus one of the 5 W's
- *Gut motility:* Signs like flatus and hunger represent recovery, and signs like emesis and distention suggest ileus and possibly even obstruction.
- *Prevention:* Ensure that your pt is walking and using the incentive spirometer to improve gut motility and avoid fever from atelectasis and DVTs.

P **Management includes antibiotics, pain control, IV fluids, and supportive care.**

Antibiotics:

Acute appy: Start a second-generation cephalosporin for 24 hrs postop.
Perf'd appy: Cover for all potential organisms in the colonic flora:
- Gram-positive (Enterococcus)
- Aerobic gram-negative coliforms
- Anaerobic organisms

Traditionally, ampicillin, gentamicin, and metronidazole are used. Broad-spectrum single agents like piperacillin-tazobactam, ticarcillin-clavulanate, or carbapenems may also be used.
Perf'd appys should be on antibiotics for at least 5 days postop and longer if the pt is still febrile.

Narcotics are the key to pain control.

Acute appys: Most need <1 day of morphine and then a few days of acetaminophen with codeine by mouth.
Perf'd appys: Usually need morphine by patient-controlled analgesia for several days.

IV fluids

All appys should have increased rate of fluid intravenously, usually starting at twice maintenance rate, and decreasing to 1.5 times maintenance. When the pt tolerates diet, without vomiting, the IV may be hep locked.

Other supportive care

Pts should be given incentive spirometry and encouraged to use it 10 times per hour while awake to prevent atelectasis.

S

How is the baby doing since his or her surgery?

Allows the parent to tell you all of their concerns regarding the postoperative period.

Ask the parents if they think the baby is in any pain.

Pyloromyotomies are small surgeries with small incisions and are often performed in <20 minutes; however, even with a small upper abdominal incision, parents will often perceive pain in their child.

Is the baby vomiting at all?

It is good to reassess the chief complaint and address any concerns the parents may have.

How is the baby tolerating the new feeding schedule?

The new feeding schedule (see below) can be initiated on the first postoperative day. It is an important assessment of the success of the surgery. Asking this question is an important follow-up to the last question. Even if the pt is not vomiting, he or she may not be ready to eat yet.

O

Check the baby's vital signs.

Tachycardia (HR > 160 in this age group) may indicate pain.

The baby should be afebrile, with normal respirations and blood pressure.

Check the baby's intake and output to make sure he or she is tolerating feeds, receiving enough IV fluids, and producing urine.

The baby's ins and outs should be balanced, with the intake being slightly greater than the output. If the total fluid output is small (<1 cc/kg/hr), consider giving an IV fluid bolus of 10–20 cc/kg of normal saline over 1 hr.

Check to see if the pt is tolerating the new feeding schedule. Emesis should be recorded.

Perform a general PE.

Do a focused exam unless the pt is symptomatic. A comprehensive exam was done on admission, and things like red reflex, testicular exam are unlikely to change.

Lungs: Rales or rhonchi may represent aspiration during surgery or postoperatively.

Heart: Heart murmur should be absent. Murmur may represent significant blood loss, which is highly unlikely with this kind of surgery.

Capillary refill: Should be less than 2 seconds because this pt should be well hydrated.

Now gently examine the abdomen. Check the wound.

The wound should be approximately 1.5 to 2 cm long in the epigastrium and clean. There should be no surrounding erythema or discharge from the wound. These signs may represent the beginnings of an infection.

Gently palpate the abdomen in an area away from the wound. It should not be distended or exquisitely tender. The baby may not even cry. Distention and exquisite tenderness should make you think of peritoneal inflammation.

Blood should be checked at least once postoperatively for a CBC and a Chem 7.

Again, the CBC should confirm minimal blood loss. There should be virtually no change in hemoglobin or hematocrit levels since admission.

The Chem 7 should have normalized. On admission, the baby can have some severe metabolic derangements, including alkalosis, hypokalemia, and hypochloremia. The BUN-to-creatinine ratio may have been greater than 20:1. With hydration, these numbers should return to normal.

If aspiration is suspected, a chest x-ray should be obtained.

A Status post-pyloromyotomy, postop day _____.

Your assessment should also mention the resolution of metabolic derangements and how the pt is doing with feeds.

Also watch for complications of the surgery, such as wound infection, peritonitis, postop fever, and recurrence of the original problem (rare).

P Begin refeeding the pt on the first postoperative day. He or she should be hungry.

Feeding should begin with an electrolyte solution such as Pedialyte. Start with only 5 cc.

If the pt tolerates this without emesis, 10 cc of Pedialyte may be given 2 hrs later.

If there is still no emesis, you may switch to 10 cc of half-strength formula 2 hrs later.

This may be increased to 15 cc 2 hrs later.

If the pt tolerates 15 cc of half-strength formula, you may now switch to full-strength formula. Repeat 15 cc.

Now, every 2 hrs the amount may be increased: 20 cc, then 30 cc, then 45 cc, and finally 60 cc. Once the pt tolerates 60 cc, feed regularly every 3 hrs.

If the pt has emesis with any of the doses of feed, feeds should be held for 4 hrs and then restarted at the last tolerated dose.

Stop IV fluids when feeds are tolerated.

Control pain with minimal amounts of intravenous narcotics. Morphine sulfate is the drug of choice.

Morphine can be given 0.1 mg/kg q2–4h prn for pain. Remember that the disadvantage of giving it is that it decreases gut motility and may worsen the recovery time.

Once the pt is tolerating regular feeds of formula or breast milk, and pain is not an issue, pt may be discharged.

There should be follow-up in a surgery clinic to check the wound and remove sutures as needed, and follow-up with a general pediatrician at the regular 2-month visit.

Does the pt have any pain? If so, where and how much does it hurt on a scale of 1 to 10?
Make sure that if your pt has pain, the etiology is discovered and the pain is controlled.

Can the pt wiggle or move his or her toes/fingers?
If the child is unable to move the toes/fingers of the cast limb and this is a new problem, this may signify neurologic damage or compartment syndrome (see below).

Can the pt feel his or her toes/fingers?
If the pt cannot feel the toes/fingers or has abnormal sensation, check for other signs of compartment syndrome.

Have the pt's toes/fingers changed color or do they feel numb or cold?
If the fingers or toes are turning blue or black, or they feel unusually numb or cold, check for pulses proximally. If they are diminished or nonpalpable, emergently notify the orthopedist and possibly vascular surgeon.

Has the pt been using the incentive spirometer?
Use of the incentive spirometer will decrease the incidence of atelectasis and possibly of postoperative pneumonia, so encourage its use.

O Examine the pt
Perform a good general PE.

Look at the vitals for any worrisome signs.
Infection: Fever could be a sign of infection.

If the fever spike is near surgery, consider the postsurgical causes of fever mnemonic: five W's =
- *W*ind (atelectasis)   - *W*ater (UTI)   - *W*ound (wound
- *W*onder drugs (drug fever)   - *W*alking (DVT)   infection)

With that in mind, get the appropriate workup. Check a chest x-ray, get urine and blood cultures, and wound cultures if appropriate.
Internal bleeding: Tachycardia can be a sign of nervousness, pain, or worse, hypovolemia. If tachycardia occurs, monitor it closely. If it persists and pain is not the cause, consider giving an IV fluid bolus. If the bolus improves the tachycardia, consider the possibility that the pt is still bleeding. Pts can bleed into places such as the abdomen, thigh, chest, or subgaleal space with little outward sign of the problem except persistent tachycardia. If you suspect this, notify the resident immediately.
Pulmonary embolus: Tachycardia, with or without hypoxia and nervousness could suggest a pulmonary embolus from fat or clot. If the suspicion is high enough, get a spiral CT scan of the chest with contrast. Call the orthopedic surgeon before starting heparin or other anticoagulants.

Look at the digits distal to the fracture, cast, or splint for signs of compartment syndrome.
These are icy cold, *P*allor, *P*aresthesias (tingling or abnormal sensation), *P*ulselessness, or especially severe *P*ain with passive movement of the toes or fingers of the affected limb.
• Mnemonic = 4P's. See Limb Trauma p. 120.

Look for signs of infection.
Look for cellulitis (warm, red, swollen, tender skin) or purulent discharge near any
hardware. Monitor carefully for possible development of osteomyelitis. Check an
x-ray (or MRI if clinical suspicion is high enough) of the affected limb for disruption
of the cortex or soft tissue swelling.

 Status post _____, postop day _____
Assess for pain control
See Pain Control p. 132.

Assess for compartment syndrome.
Increased pressure is usually caused by inflammation and swelling in a space enclosed
by fascial planes. When the pressure exceeds that of local arterial blood flow, ischemia
results. Evaluate carefully and remember the 4 P's (see above).

Assess for internal bleeding.
Look carefully for:
- Persistent tachycardia   - Drop in hematocrit   - Pallor
- Hypotension   - Local swelling

Assess for infection.
It is important to rule in or out osteomyelitis because the treatment for this is chronic
antibiotics, and the longer it goes unrecognized, the harder it is to eradicate.

**Consider offering physical therapy (PT) and/or occupational therapy
(OT).**
Usually the answer to this offer is yes. Call PT and OT to see if they can offer any help
with the pt's rehabilitation.

P **Control the pt's pain**
See Pain Control p. 132.

Treat compartment syndrome if it is present.
The treatment is to surgically release the pressure by opening the space enclosed by
fascia = fasciotomy. If this needs to be done emergently, notify the orthopedic
surgeon.

Resuscitate the pt and control/stop internal bleeding if it is present.
If you suspect internal bleeding, stabilize/resuscitate the pt with normal saline boluses
20 mL/kg up to 3 times, then start transfusing blood. In the meantime, emergently
contact the surgeon for possible surgery to achieve hemostasis.

**If you suspect infection, obtain blood cultures, x-rays, MRI, and other
studies as appropriate.**
Based on the results of the workup for fever, x-ray, U/A, blood, urine, or wound
culture, treat the infection appropriately. If osteomyelitis is diagnosed (often on
MRI), the pt will need long-term treatment (at least 6 weeks) with antibiotics and
possibly even surgical insertion of antibiotic pellets into the bone for better local
delivery of the antibiotic.

Prepare pt for discharge.
Keep the pain well-controlled. Get the pt as active as possible within the constraints of
the injury. Consult PT and OT for tips and advice on how to do this, as well as
exercises and strategies the pt can use to make the transition from hospital to home.

VI

Pediatric Intensive Care Unit

S The PICU is a special place. It is different from other pediatric areas in many respects, including notes. The format of the PICU note is organized a little differently from the typical SOAP format, but in reality it is only a slight variation.

The ICU note is organized by system and within each system. Although it is often not explicitly written, there is a SOAP structure:

(**S**) Any subjective complaints related to that symptom

(**O**) Vital signs, PE, labs, and studies that pertain specifically to the system

(**A**) System-based assessment that synthesizes the above information into a system-based problem list and an assessment of the status of each

(**P**) Make a clear plan for each problem identified in the assessment. Often the assessment and plan section are combined into one A/P section.

An example of the Note format is as follows:

Time & Date: 11/24/3 at 13:56 (Use 24-hr time to avoid confusion about a.m. or p.m.)

ID: James is a 6-yr-old boy Hospital Day 7 with

1. Severe cerebral palsy
2. Seizure disorder
3. Bronchopulmonary dysplasia
4. Pneumonia
5. Sepsis resolving

Medications:
Dopamine Drip at 1 mcg/kg/min
Ceftriaxone 500 mg IV q6h Day 7/10
Phenobarbitol 120 mg per g-tube qd
Ranitidine 100 mg per g-tube bid
Acetaminophen 300 mg per g-tube
prn pain & T > 38

Hardware (and how old it is): Central Line placed 5 days ago, Foley last changed yesterday.

IV Fluid (composition and rate): e.g., D5$^{1}/_{2}$ NS at 40 cc/hr.

Diet: NPO with Tube feeds at 20 cc/hr.

Neuro:

(S) Note whether there are any specific complaints related to pain, balance, or other potentially neuro-mediated symptoms.

(O) Note the pain score, Glasgow Coma Score, mental status, neuro exam (motor, reflexes, sensory, coordination, gait) and any labs or studies like LP results, CT of brain, EEG, etc.

(A/P) Record your assessment of the pt's neuro status (mental status, pain control, etc.) and whether there has been any change (improvement or worsening) since the last note. Also record any plans you have to adjust pain meds or obtain studies like MRI of the brain.

Resp:

(S) Subjective complaints such as shortness of breath and cough

(O) Note vital signs, vent settings, PE findings in the lungs, chest x-rays, ABG results, sputum quality/cultures, etc.

(A/P) Assess the pt's respiratory status and any plans you have, such as weaning from the ventilator or placing a tracheostomy.

CV:

(S) Subjective cardiovascular complaints or problems such as chest pain or palpitations

(O) Note heart rate, BP, and cardiovascular exam.

(A/P) Assess pt's cardiovascular status and comment on any plans you may have, such as weaning off pressors or placing a Swan-Ganz catheter to assess volume status.

FEN/GI:

(S) Subjective complaints, eating and stooling, last BM

(O) Record the ins and outs, the abdominal exam, the labs pertaining to electrolytes (Chem 7) and nutrition (e.g., albumin, prealbumin, LFTs), food intake, and any studies pertaining to this system, such as KUB or CT of the abdomen.

(A/P) Assess the pt's fluid, electrolyte, and nutrition status and make plans to continue with the current plan or replace electrolytes, advance diet, etc.

Renal/GU:

(S) Record any subjective complaints pertaining to the renal or genitourinary systems.

(O) Record the genital exam if it was done and note urine output in cc/kg/hr. Also record any labs like BUN and Creatinine or studies like renal U/S or VCUG.

(A/P) Assess renal function and calculate urine output, and explain any changes in the plan as a result of this data.

Heme/ID:

(S) Any subjective data pertaining to Heme or ID

(O) Record whether there was fever, pallor on exam, and any labs like CBC, and all microbiology that is completed or pending.

(A/P) Assess the hematologic and infectious status of the pt. Make decisions to transfuse or start or change antimicrobial therapy.

Other Systems: Endocrine, Derm, Musculoskeletal, Ob/Gyn, Psych, Oncology, or whatever topics contain the pt's remaining problems.

(S)

(O)

(A/P)

ICU: Discuss topics particular to the ICU, such as prophylaxis with H_2 blocker for stress ulcers and leg squeezers for DVT.

Code Status: Full Code (or whatever the pt and their family has decided)

Social: Discuss any issues related to the social situation of the child. Issues related to child abuse, neglect, or even just comments on updating the parents should be noted here.

(Finally, be sure to sign your note and write your name and pager number legibly next to your signature.)

S **How is the child currently different from his or her baseline?**

Obtain baseline so mental retardation is not misdiagnosed as altered mental status (AMS).

Characterize mental state:
- Awake, alert, and oriented × 4 (person, place, time, and situation)
- Lethargic (sleepy)　　- Obtunded (wakes but falls right back to sleep)
- Confused　　　　　　- Comatose

When did this start? Did the onset occur gradually or suddenly?

Gradual onset suggests psychosis, dementia, or encephalopathy.

Rapid onset is more consistent with delirium, intoxication, or intracranial bleed.

Has there been gradual withdrawal from family/friends over the past few months?

This can be another indication of onset of psychosis, especially in adolescents.

Is there any history of head trauma?

Trauma and intracranial bleed can cause AMS.

Does the child have any chronic medical conditions?

Ask specifically about diabetes, seizure disorder, renal problems, and psychiatric problems.

Has the child been ill recently?

Septic shock can present as AMS and is often preceded by some type of illness.

Encephalitis may present after a viral prodrome.

Is there a possibility that the pt could be intoxicated?

In adolescents, parents may be unaware of the pt's substance abuse until the first ER visit.

Children and toddlers may have gotten into household medications such as oral hypoglycemics.

Is there a history of colicky abdominal pain?

Intussusception can have a component of AMS in later stages.

O **Begin by checking the pt's vital signs.**

Vital signs may help indicate the etiology of AMS:
- Fever indicates infectious etiology such as encephalitis, sepsis, or meningitis.
- Tachycardia may indicate alcohol intoxication or hypoglycemia.
- Bradycardia and bradypnea can indicate opiate intoxication.
- Hypotension is consistent with late-stage shock of any type.
- Bradycardia with hypertension and abnormal breathing is Cushing's triad, a late sign of increased intracranial pressure.

Rapidly obtain a fingerstick glucose.

Hypoglycemia is a potentially dangerous cause of AMS; it is easily treated and so should be diagnosed as quickly as possible. Normal range for glucose is between 70 and 110.

Age of the pt

Certain diagnoses are more common in certain age groups. Intussusception is more common in infancy, whereas psychosis and intoxication are more common in adolescents.

Assess the Glasgow Coma Score (GCS). (See Table 8.)
Perform a general PE.

Pinpoint pupils are consistent with opiate intoxication.

Unequal pupils may indicate an expanding intracranial mass or bleed.
Blinking, staring, lip-smacking, or abnormal movements may indicate seizure.
Nuchal rigidity may indicate meningoencephalitis.
Rales on lung exam may indicate pneumonia, a source of sepsis.
An infant with a tender, sausage-shaped abdominal mass may indicate intussusception.

Place a Foley catheter and send urine for a U/A and a urine toxicology screen.
Intoxication may be diagnosed in this manner, as can some renal conditions.

Send blood for CBC with differential, Chem 7 with a calcium, and serum toxicology panel.
The chemistries will reveal renal failure or electrolyte disturbances. CBC may suggest
  sepsis.
Alcohol or other intoxication may be diagnosed by the serum toxicology.

Obtain a CT scan of the head and, if nondiagnostic, obtain an MRI.
These should help to diagnose intracranial bleed or mass.

If CT is normal, a lumbar puncture is indicated.
Increased WBC count indicates meningitis.
- Bacterial meningitis is suggested by neutrophil predominance.
- Viral meningoencephalitis is more likely to have lymphocytosis.
- Herpes encephalitis has lymphocytosis and RBCs with xanthochromia on an
  atraumatic tap.

Altered Mental Status
Any time the thought processes function in a manner different from normal

Differential diagnosis

A good mnemonic for the differential of AMS is AEIOU TIPS:

- Alcohol intoxication	- Encephalitis	- Endocrinopathy
- Electrolyte abnormalities	- Insulin overdose	- Intussusception
- Opiate intoxication	- Uremia	- Trauma
- Infection	- Psychosis	- Seizures

P **Plan depends on etiology, but always intubate if GCS <8.**
Alcohol intoxication: Provide supportive care and assessment of how the child obtained
  the alcohol.
Encephalitis: If herpes, start acyclovir. For a suspected bacterial infection, give
  antibiotics.
Endocrinopathy: Thyroid storm is treated with beta-blockers, a thiourea, iodine, and
  steroids. Adrenal insufficiency is treated with corticosteroids.
Electrolyte abnormalities: Replace lytes as needed.
Insulin overdose: Treat with glucose and then reassess insulin regimen and diet.
Intussusception: Treat with enema (barium or air) or surgical reduction if enema fails.
Uremia: Treat with dialysis and then a workup to discover why it worsened.
Trauma/intracranial bleed: Treat with measures like mannitol until surgical
  decompression.
Infection/Sepsis: Treat with broad-spectrum antibiotics.
Psychosis: Can be treated with antipsychotics.
Seizures: Can be treated with antiepileptics like benzodiazepines.

S **Does the pt have a history of previous intubation?**
If so, pt may have chronic respiratory issues and could be a more difficult intubation.

Does the pt have any acute or chronic medical problems?
Consider the impact and implications on management and workup of acute problems
  such as:

          - Altered mental status (AMS)   - Pneumonia
          - Asthma   - Croup
It is also important to consider other preexisting conditions, such as:
          - Chronic lung disease   - Neurologic impairment   - Heart disease
          - Liver disease   - Kidney disease

Did the pt receive any medicines for pain recently?
Overdoses of pain meds are a common cause of iatrogenic respiratory failure.

O **Begin with assessing responsiveness and the pt's ABCs (airway, breathing, circulation). These should all be done almost simultaneously.**
Assess responsiveness quickly and confirm that the pt is unarousable.
Airway: Position pt on back in the sniffing position (with chin slightly up). Examine
  oropharynx for obstruction.
Breathing: Look, listen, and feel for breath from the pt. If the pt is not breathing, place
  an oral airway and use the bag-valve-mask by holding the mask firmly to the pt's face
  while squeezing the bag completely about once every 3 to 5 seconds.
Circulation: Check for peripheral and central pulses.

Quickly call for O$_2$, IV, and monitor as if it is one word.
O$_2$: Supplemental oxygen and prepare to intubate.
IV: Place two large-bore IVs and obtain the following labs: glucose, stat electrolytes,
  toxicology screen, and an arterial blood gas (ABG).
Monitor vital signs, rhythm, and pulse oximetry.
Review the vital signs and PE for signs of respiratory distress: subcostal retractions,
  tachypnea, tachycardia, hypoxia, suprasternal retractions, abdominal breathing,
  cyanosis, wheezing, AMS with Glasgow Coma Score (GCS) < 8, nasal flaring,
  grunting, rhonchi, poor air entry on lung exam.
Review the chart and information from your monitor.

Interpret the ABG.
Remember the order and normal values:
  pH/pCO$_2$/pO$_2$/HCO$_3$/oxygen Sat
  7.40/40/>85/25/>97%

Remember the relationship between pH, pCO$_2$, and HCO$_3$:
  • pH $\propto$ HCO$_3$/pCO$_2$. In other words, pH is proportional to bicarb (metabolic =
    kidneys) over pCO$_2$ (respiratory = lungs).

Look at the pH and decide if this is an acidemia or an alkalemia.
Look at the pCO$_2$ and decide if this is primarily a respiratory or metabolic problem.
  Based on the proportionality listed above, in order for it to be a primary respiratory
  disorder, a low pH (<7.4) should be caused by a high pCO$_2$ and a high pH should be
  caused by a low pCO$_2$. If this is not the case, then it is a primary metabolic process.
  Hypoxia can be tolerated down to a pO$_2$ of ~70 mm Hg and a sat of >94%.

A **Review the causes of acute respiratory failure:**
Pulmonary: Asthma, croup, epiglottitis, foreign body, pneumonia, acute respiratory
  distress syndrome (ARDS)

Neurologic: AMS with decreased or absent respiratory drive
Cardiovascular: Heart failure, arrhythmia, or anemia

Reasons to intubate

The decision to intubate is often clinical and can be based on the need for airway
protection as a result of:

- Impending airway obstruction   - Lung pathology   - Heart pathology
- Inability to maintain ventilation   - Low GCS   - Absent gag
- Decreased respiratory drive

Often, an ABG will be drawn to help with this decision.

ABG results consistent with respiratory failure are:

pO_2 < 50 or oxygen saturation < 75% on 60% FiO_2
pCO_2 > 50 (with a pH < 7.30) or > 40 (with respiratory fatigue)

P Intubate. Mnemonic: PS ALAN B SIC

*P*osition pt on a back board with a neck roll under the shoulders.
*S*elect size of endotracheal tube (ETT) and laryngoscope blade (with Broeslow tape).
Calculate the size of ETT needed, with ETT = (Age/4) + 4.
Place the *S*tylet in the ETT.
Draw up *A*tropine 0.02 mg/kg if the pt is <5 yrs old in case of severe vagal response
to intubation caused by high vagal tone in the younger ages.
If you suspect increased intracranial pressure, give *L*idocaine 1 mg/kg.
Give *A*tivan 0.05 mg/kg IV to sedate.
Give *N*orcuron 0.1 mg/kg IV to paralyze. Wait until the pt is paralyzed about
2–5 minutes.
Use the *B*ag-valve-mask to hyperventilate the pt.
Then apply cricoid pressure (*S*ellick maneuver) to prevent emesis and to align the
airway.
*I*ntubate. Make sure that you see the ETT go through the vocal cords.
*C*onfirm tube placement and secure it in place.

Choose initial ventilator settings.

FiO_2 of 100%. Wean quickly to the lowest possible level to avoid O_2 free radical damage.
Set respiratory rate at normal for age or half of the spontaneous rate.
Set PEEP to 5 and choose ventilator mode:

- Synchronized intermittent mandatory ventilation requires a set peak inspiratory
  pressure of about 20 cm H_2O.
- Pressure-regulated volume control requires a set Vt (tidal volume) of about
  7–10 cc/kg.

Vent Changes:

To change the pH and pCO_2, you need to change Minute Ventilation.

- Minute Ventilation = Tidal Volume × Respiratory Rate (MV = Vt × RR).

To correct acidosis (↑pH or ↓pCO_2), increase either Vt or RR to blow off CO_2.
To correct hypoxia, there are two options:

- Increase FiO_2 if the cause is:
  - Diffusion abnormality (interstitial lung disease)
  - Ventilation/perfusion mismatch (asthma, pulmonary hypertension or
    embolus)
- Increase positive end expiratory pressure for a pulmonary right-to-left shunt
  (ARDS, edema, or pneumonia).

S   **For any pt in shock, aggressive rapid stabilization should come before history. After or while the child is being stabilized, the history may be taken from the parent. Obtain a history of the infection leading up to the current septic shock.**

Giving a history during resuscitation/stabilization will give the parents something to do and make them feel useful where they would otherwise feel helpless.

The history will help you determine the source of sepsis and direct your choice of therapy.

Does the child have cancer or any other new symptoms such as bruising, bleeding, or fatigue?

Pts on chemotherapy and all leukemics before treatment are functionally immunosuppressed and are at a high risk of fulminant sepsis.

Has the child had a splenectomy? Does he or she have sickle cell disease?

Pts who have had their spleen either removed or autoinfarcted (as in sickle cell disease) will have difficulty mounting a response to encapsulated organisms, such as:

- *Streptococcus pneumoniae*   - *Haemophilus influenzae*   - *Neisseria meningitidis*

Is the child taking any medications?

Immunosuppressants, such as prednisone, imuran, and cyclosporin, can increase the risk of sepsis.

Some medications can cause neutropenia:

- Antipsychotics   - Penicillins
- Sulfa-based antibiotics   - Anticonvulsants

Does the child have any chronic medical conditions?

- Diabetes mellitus   - AIDS   - Congenital immune deficiency

O   **Start by checking pt's vital signs, including oxygen saturation.**

Vital signs consistent with septic shock are tachycardia, tachypnea, fever, and hypotension.

Bradycardia with hypotension is an ominous sign.

Check to see if the child has an appropriate mental status.

Altered mental status is an important clinical sign of systemic organ dysfunction.

Lack of fight or cry during the exam or procedure is a notable abnormality.

Perform a rapid but complete physical assessment.

Rales on lung exam may indicate pneumonia.

Heart murmur could mean endocarditis.

Nuchal rigidity indicates meningitis.

Exquisite abdominal tenderness to palpation suggests an intestinal source:

- Perforation   - Intussusception
- Appendicitis   - Neutropenic colitis (typhlitis)

Check capillary refill: 1 to 2 seconds is normal. Septic shock should have prolongation of greater than 3 seconds, or an instant flash of returning blood, depending on the phase.

Feel for peripheral pulses and, if they are not detectable, check for central pulses. If they are present (skin is likely to be cool and mottled), this suggests a systolic blood pressure of 60 mm Hg.

Place a Foley catheter to measure urine output (be sure to send U/A and UCx).

Monitor ins and outs. If urine output < 1 cc/kg/hr, consider either hypovolemia or renal failure.

Order a CBC with differential, culture, and a blood gas.

pH, pCO_2, bicarb, anion gap, and lactate are important indicators of hypoperfusion severity.

Check WBC, differential, and band count to assess signs of infection or neutropenia.

Culture before antibiotics (blood, urine, sputum, and, if indicated, CSF).

If a Swann-Ganz catheter is placed, the vascular parameters can be evaluated.

Both systemic vascular resistance and pulmonary vascular wedge pressure are decreased in septic shock. Early on, cardiac output is increased, and then decreases later as shock worsens.

Septic shock

Shock is a state of underperfusion of end organs, with evidence of end organ dysfunction.

The massive inflammatory response to the circulating pathogen (usually a Gram-negative organism) causes vasodilation, cardiac dysfunction, and impaired tissue oxygen extraction.

Fever with neutropenia ([(% Segs + % Bands) x WBC] <500)

Very high risk of fulminant sepsis. Treat aggressively even if fever is the only symptom.

Differential diagnosis of fever with shock

The following should all be treated as septic shock until it is ruled out:

- Intracranial bleed	- Intoxication	- Burns
- Heat shock	- Myocarditis	

P **Give up to three 20 cc/kg boluses of normal saline (NS) IV.**

Fluid resuscitation should be with isotonic crystalloid (normal saline) in IV boluses (or intraosseously if an IV cannot be established) until the pt responds with decreasing heart rate and increasing urine output.

After three boluses of NS, if the pt needs further boluses, a colloid such as blood or albumin should be used.

This is to avoid volume overload and continued decrease in oncotic pressure.

If there is not sufficient response to the boluses, start dopamine at 5 mcg/kg/min and titrate to an appropriate systolic blood pressure.

If dopamine is ineffective, try dobutamine, norepinephrine, and finally epinephrine drips as needed for pressor effects.

Start broad-spectrum antibiotics until cultures reveal organism sensitivity.

Broad-spectrum antibiotics include:

- An antipseudomonal aminoglycoside (amikacin or tobramycin)
- Plus a third-generation cephalosporin (ceftazidime or cefotaxime)

Alternative regimens include:

- Carbapenems or antipseudomonal penicillins or a fourth-generation cephalosporin

Most critical care physicians recommend that if the pt has septic shock, intubation and mechanical ventilation are important adjuncts to therapy.

Diagnose and treat the etiology of the sepsis!

S **Initial management is to stabilize the child and then take the history. Does the child have a history of any heart problems?**

Most children who experience cardiogenic shock will have some kind of cardiac disease history. Most parents will know and immediately tell you about a history of:
- Congenital heart defects   - Heart surgeries   - Trips to the cardiologist

If there is a history of heart disease, has pt been taking all of his or her medications?

If pt is reliant on medical therapy, a failure in compliance may set up cardiogenic shock.

Has the child had any history of loss of consciousness or palpitations with exercise?

Syncope or palpitations with exercise may indicate a cardiac conduction defect (long QT syndrome or Wolff-Parkinson-White) or an outlet obstruction (idiopathic hypertrophic subaortic stenosis). Either may cause an arrhythmia, which may lead to cardiogenic shock.

Has the child had any recent illnesses or infections?

A recent viral illness may have been a prodrome for a myocarditis, usually caused by coxsackie viruses. With myocarditis, cardiac function can decrease rapidly.

A history of a throat infection, followed by rash and migratory arthritis, may indicate acute rheumatic fever, which can cause a myocarditis or a pericarditis with tamponade from effusion.

A history of Kawasaki disease or just high fever, rashes, conjunctivitis, and mouth lesions can cause both myocarditis and ectasias of the coronary arteries that can lead to a myocardial infarction (MI).

Has there been any history of recent chest trauma?

In the case that there may have been a recent car accident or a blow to the chest, pericardial bleeding may result, causing a cardiac tamponade. A bruise should be visible.

Has the child just come out of surgery?

Cardiogenic shock is a rare postoperative complication.

O **Check the vital signs.**

Bradycardia and hypotension: The heart may be failing to meet the body's metabolic needs.

If there is no pulse, call a Code Blue and follow the **Pediatric Advanced Life Support (PALS)** protocol.

Place an electrical rhythm monitor on the chest and obtain a 12-lead ECG.

Cardiogenic shock may present with several different rhythms (sinus tachycardia is common).

Slow heart rate may be sinus bradycardia or an AV block.

No pulse is likely to be asystole, but it may also be ventricular tachycardia or fibrillation.

Pulseless electrical activity (PEA): No pulse, but a rhythm is present on the monitor. Of the many causes of PEA, one should consider cardiac tamponade in children.

Supraventricular tachycardia: P-waves will not be present and rate will be extremely rapid, usually faster than can be accounted for by sinus tachycardia alone. If the rate is so fast that the ventricles do not have time to fill between contractions, cardiogenic shock may occur.

Perform a PE.

Look for altered mental status and cool mottling of the skin with poor capillary refill times.

Cardiogenic shock has poor forward blood flow, so look for signs of venous congestion:

- Rales occur bilaterally on pulmonary auscultation as blood backs up into the lungs.
- The jugular veins may be visible.
- The liver will likely be palpable and may even be pulsatile.
- Children rarely present with edema secondary to cardiac dysfunction.

Heart exam:

- Rhythm: Fast, slow, or nonexistent
- Murmur: May indicate a congenital heart defect.
- S_3: A low-pitched tone after S_2, common in cardiogenic shock.
- S_4: A heart sound preceding S_1, somewhat less common.

Place a Foley catheter.

Urine output will be decreased in shock.

Obtain an echocardiogram.

An U/S of the heart is helpful to see ejection fraction (a measure of heart function), congenital heart defects, and pericardial fluid that may be causing tamponade.

A   Cardiogenic shock

Occurs when the pump fails to meet the metabolic needs of the rest of the body, usually including itself. When tissues do not receive their proper oxygen supply, they tend to make lactic acid. Acidosis worsens cardiac function. A downward spiral occurs.

Some of the possible causes are:

- Myocarditis	- Endocarditis	- Cardiomyopathy	
- Tamponade	- Arrhythmia	- Valvular stenosis	- MI

Consider other causes of shock:

Neurogenic: Severe pain, stroke, intracranial bleed
Hypovolemic: Bleeding, dehydration, third spacing
Anaphylactic: Envenomations, transfusion, contrast reactions
Vascular obstruction: Massive pulmonary embolus, pneumothorax, excessive positive end expiratory pressure
Septic: Any infection that becomes systemic

P   The initial management of shock always involves giving IV fluids, even in this case.

If the fluids are followed by worsening symptoms, IV furosemide 1 mg/kg may be given. It causes rapid urine output and thus is an afterload reducer.

Start dobutamine at 5 mcg/kg/min and titrate to effect.

Dobutamine causes improved myocardial contractility with some peripheral vasodilation.

Supraventricular tachycardias should be treated with adenosine 0.1 mg/kg IV push.

If no response, double the dose and repeat.

If the child is pulseless, call a Code Blue and follow the PALS protocols.

Is the child a diabetic? If so, has he or she been taking insulin appropriately?

Diabetic ketoacidosis (DKA) is a common presenting symptom of type I diabetes mellitus (DM).

Also occurs in type 2 DM or any diabetic who falls significantly short of insulin needs.

Is the child excessively hungry or thirsty? Is there increasing urination (how many times per night)? Has he or she been losing weight?

The classic presentation of DKA is weight loss, polyuria, polydipsia, and polyphagia.

Lack of insulin leads to decreased cellular entry of glucose (cellular hypoglycemia) and increased serum glucose.

When serum glucose > 180, glycosuria begins causing an osmotic diuresis, which leads to the *polyuria,* which leads to dehydration, causing *polydipsia* (excessive thirst).

Cellular hypoglycemia stimulates excessive hunger (*polyphagia*).

The dehydration and increased metabolic state contribute to the *weight loss.*

Does the child have abdominal pain, nausea, or vomiting?

These are common symptoms of DKA that can be caused by the acidosis of DKA. However, because comorbid diagnoses such as appendicitis and pancreatitis can trigger DKA, such conditions should be carefully considered and ruled out.

O Look carefully for signs that help confirm the diagnosis.

Most children with DKA are dehydrated. Look for signs of this in:

- Tachycardia   - Dry mucus membranes
- Skin tenting   - Delayed cap refill

Look for signs of hypotension, altered mental status, or respiratory compromise.

Signs that aggressive intervention and ICU transfer should be pursued are:

- Kussmaul's respirations   - Altered mental status   - Hypotension

Perform a focused exam and studies to rule out other causes of abdominal pain and AMS:

DKA often appears with abdominal pain and AMS, but carefully rule out:

- Appendicitis   - Drug overdose
- Infections   - Other diagnoses

Check a fingerstick glucose, a blood gas, a stat Chem 7, and a U/A.

A high glucose should prompt rapid rehydration.

A blood gas will tell the current pH and pCO_2, from which you can assess the acid–base status.

A stat Chem 7 will show all of the electrolytes that must be followed.

The U/A must show both glucose and ketones to make the diagnosis.

A Diabetic Ketoacidosis

No other conditions cause hyperglycemia, ketonuria, and acidosis together in the same pt.

Make a flow sheet of the important labs (see Table 12).

Check labs every hour at first and then every 2 to 4 hrs as the lab values improve.

pH less than 7.4 is acidemia; less than 7.2 is considered severe.

Na decreases due to high serum glucose. Corrected Na = Na + [(Ser Glucose – 100)/100] × 1.6.

While initial K values may be in the normal range, keep in mind that prolonged

diuresis, volume contraction, and a lack of insulin will combine to falsely elevate the value. Total body stores of K are actually low and will need to be replaced.
Cl is invariably the first number to normalize and then reach supernormal levels with increased treatment. It is the number initially responsible for "closing" the anion gap.
HCO_3 represents the level of metabolic acidosis in the body.
Anion gap (AG): Follow carefully until it is <15. Calculate AG by subtracting the bicarbonate and the chloride from the sodium. If AG > 15, the gap is "open," representing the presence of organic acids (ketones). Recovery phase begins when the gap "closes" (AG < 15).
Glucose: Follow serum glucose, because when it gets below 300, dextrose should be added to the IV fluids as D5 to prevent iatrogenic hypoglycemia.

Table 12 Lab Flowsheet

Time	pH	Na	K	Cl	HCO₃	AG	Gluc	UrKet	UrGluc
02:33	7.20	131	3.9	96	11	24	622	+	>1000

P **Treat with rehydration, insulin, and electrolyte replacement.**
Repeat boluses of 10–20 cc NS/kg until signs of hypotension or poor perfusion resolve.
The pathology here is from dehydration secondary to long-term osmotic diuresis.

Start an insulin drip IV at 0.1 U/kg/hr.
Insulin is the only effective treatment for DKA because lack of insulin is the etiology.

After the boluses finish, start a 1/2 NS IV at 1.5–2 times maintenance.
Because of initial dehydration and ongoing losses, aggressive IVF therapy is required.

Add 40 mEq KCl/L to the IVF when the child begins to make urine.
The polyuria and diuresis of DKA causes an overall lack of K.
Initially, serum K is falsely elevated as a result of lack of insulin, which facilitates K's entry into cells. When insulin therapy begins, the K will again enter the cells and cause hypokalemia.
To avoid potentially lethal arrhythmias, start K early.

Add D5 (5% Dextrose) to the IVF when serum glucose <300.
This prevents hypoglycemia and reduces the ongoing catabolism.

Check electrolytes (K, Phos, Mg, Ca) every 2 to 4 hrs and replace as needed.
Electrolyte abnormalities can cause lethal sequelae such as arrhythmia, seizure, or cerebral edema.

When acidosis, high AG, low bicarb, and glycosuria all resolve, stop the insulin drip and give 0.25 U/kg of regular insulin SQ q4h until the pt begins to eat.
While the pt is not eating, this is a better regimen to avoid hypoglycemia.

When the pt begins to eat, stop the above regimen 4 hrs before breakfast and calculate and initiate an insulin regimen.
Insulin can be calculated as 0.5 U/kg/day.
- 2/3 of this should be given in the morning 30 minutes before breakfast; 1/3 short-acting insulin (such as Regular); 2/3 long-acting insulin (such as NPH)
- 1/3 in the evening; 1/2 short-acting insulin 30 minutes before dinner; 1/2 long-acting insulin at bedtime

S **What was the mechanism of head injury?**
Traumatic Brain Injury (Glasgow Coma Score $\leq$ to 8) occurs with more severe injuries:
    - Motor vehicle accident (unrestrained passenger)   - Auto versus bicycle
    - Fall from > 15 feet   - Auto versus pedestrian   - Diving injuries

Has the child been conscious at all since the event?
Epidural hematoma: Presents as a lucid interval (an initial loss of consciousness after which the pt regains consciousness and then progressively loses it again).
Diffuse axonal injury: Presents as a persistent state of unconsciousness since the event.

If there was a period of consciousness, did the child have any other symptoms?
Increasing intracranial pressure (ICP): Decreased level of consciousness with persistent vomiting and headache.
Parenchymal brain injury: Can present as seizures.

O **Check the pt's vital signs.**
Cushing's triad: Hypertension associated with bradycardia and bradypnea. A late sign of increased ICP.
Fever: Can occur with any reabsorption of blood from inside the head. Treat with antipyretics and cooling measures, such as ice packs, if over 37.5°C.

Check the pt's pupillary response.
Normal pupils should be equal, round, and reactive to light.
Impending cerebral herniation: Can present as a single dilated pupil that does not respond to light; treat as such until proven otherwise.

Rate the pt's Glasgow Coma Score (GCS) to help assess pt.
See Head Trauma p. 118 for GCS table.
The maximum score is 15, the minimum is 3.
An example of how GCS is usually recorded is $E_2M_3V_2 = GCS\ 7$.
Most pts that go to the PICU with head trauma will have a GCS of < 8.
Remember if GCS < 8, intubate.

Carefully review the head CT.
Severe head injuries tend to present on CT scan as:
- *Bleeds:* Can be epidural, subdural, subarachnoid, or intraparenchymal.
  - *Epidural hematoma:* A lentiform-shaped bleed not crossing suture lines, compressing the brain. It is arterial and usually results from rupture of the middle meningeal artery.
  - *Subdural hematoma:* A crescent-shaped bleed usually covering an entire hemisphere of the brain. This bleed is venous and results from tearing of the bridging veins. In infants, it is common in child abuse. It is associated with the highest morbidity and mortality of any bleed, despite exerting less pressure on the brain than the epidural hematoma.
  - *Subarachnoid hemorrhage:* Blood around the brain. It is usually not associated with trauma and is more often spontaneous, associated with severe headache without GCS depression. Usually caused by a bleeding arteriovenous malformation (AVM) or berry aneurysm.
  - *Intraparenchymal hemorrhage:* Bleed in the brain tissue. If small, it is called a contusion. Can cause focal or generalized neurologic deficits.
- *Shear:* Diffuse axonal injury can be severe. Seen on CT scan as generalized brain edema or tears in the white matter (rare). Common with rapid acceleration/deceleration injuries.

A **Traumatic brain injury (TBI)**
Severe head trauma with a low GCS (≤8).

Differential diagnosis (less likely if confirmed history of head trauma)
- Spontaneous rupture   - Subarachnoid hemorrhage   - Physical abuse
   of AVM   - Encephalitis/meningitis/sepsis   - Intoxications
- Hemorrhagic stroke

P **Follow the data from the ICP monitor.**
All pts with a TBI and a GCS of 8 or less should have had an ICP monitor placed in the
ER by a neurosurgeon, unless a surgical intervention was performed at that time.
- Two types of pressure monitors: a ventriculostomy and a bolt. The advantage of a
ventriculostomy is that cerebrospinal fluid (CSF) can be drained if necessary,
whereas with a bolt it cannot. However, bolts are less invasive than
ventriculostomies and less likely to cause injury.
Normal ICP is less than 20 mm Hg. If pt's ICP is not at this level, consider initiating
therapy to lower ICP.

Calculate and monitor cerebral perfusion pressure (CPP).
Monitoring and maintenance of CPP improves oxygenation of the brain parenchyma.
CPP is defined as mean arterial pressure (MAP) minus the ICP. Normal CPP is 40 to 65.
   - CPP = MAP − ICP   - MAP = (SBP + 2DBP)/3
So for a BP of 120/80 (MAP = 93), with an ICP of 20, the CPP is 73.

Keep CPP between 40 and 65 mm Hg.
If systemic blood pressure is low and the pt needs IV fluids/pressors
ICP is too high and it needs to be lowered:
- Sedate and anesthetize the pt with a benzodiazepine and then morphine sulfate.
- Elevate the head of the bed to 30 degrees.
- If the ICP monitor is a ventriculostomy, CSF may be drained to lower ICP.
- If ICP remains elevated, the pt can be paralyzed with Norcuron.
- Removal of cerebral edema fluid with a hyperosmolar solution intravenously
such as mannitol 0.25–1 g/kg can be an effective means of decreasing ICP.
- Hyperventilation until the pCO_2 decreases to between 30 and 35 mm Hg will
cause vasoconstriction of the cerebral arteries.
- If these measures are ineffective, start a pentobarbital drip to induce a coma.

CT scan can be repeated at any time to evaluate for new lesions. Any evidence of herniation requires emergent mannitol and hyperventilation.
Frequently reevaluate pt's vitals signs, PE, and GCS.

S   **What was the mechanism of injury?**

There are many different types of burns:

- *Scalding* (most frequent): 85% of all burn injuries in children. Usually <4 yrs old.
- *Flame:* 13% are flame burns.
- *Electrical and chemical:* Comprise the other 2%.

What time did the injury occur?

Suspect abuse if there is a significant delay between injury and seeking medical attention.

The first IV fluid dose should occur within the first 8 hrs after the injury.

O   **Begin by checking the pt's vital signs.**

It is common to see tachycardia and tachypnea.

Examine the burn and determine the size.

If the pt is more than 14 years old, then use:

- *The Rule of Nines:* Each of the following are 9% of the total body surface area (BSA): head, chest, upper back, lower back, abdomen, arm, front of leg, back of leg
- Perineum is 1%.

If the pt is less than 14 years old, estimate burn size using the pt's palm. An area equal to the palm from the wrist crease to finger creases = 1% BSA.

Now determine the severity of the burn by thickness:

Superficial epidermal burns (formerly 1st degree): Characterized by simple reddening and warmth of the skin. These burns blanche with pressure like a typical sunburn.

Superficial partial-thickness burns (2nd degree): Blisters/bullae, red, moist, extremely painful

Deep partial-thickness burns (2nd degree): The tissue is dark red or yellow-white and there is decreased sensation secondary to destruction of nerve endings.

Full-thickness burns (3rd and 4th degree): Involve the subcutaneous tissues. They appear white or charred, with eschar. Thrombosed vessels may be visible.

Finally, determine whether the burn appears accidental versus purposeful.

The following are suspicious for abuse:

- Stocking-glove burns of the hands and feet
- Full-thickness burns of the perineum, buttock, or trunk
- Burns in patterns such as a triangle (clothes iron) or circular (cigar or cigarette burn).

In the case of flame burns, examine the mouth for evidence of inhalation injury.

Pts who have inhalation injury have a risk of airway edema, pulmonary edema, or pneumonitis, which can be life-threatening.

Inhalation injury can be recognized by evidence of burning of the face, wheezing or rales (especially around the mouth or nose), and soot-tinged sputum.

Draw blood for baseline electrolytes, creatinine kinase (CK), and renal function.

Follow electrolytes: Burn injuries can cause a significant amount of fluid shifting/loss.

Check a CK to rule out rhabdomyolysis if the burns are deep enough to involve muscle.

A **Burn injury. Specify minor, moderate, or major:**
Minor: Almost all superficial burns, and any partial-thickness burns < 10% BSA
Moderate: Partial-thickness burns 10% to 20% of BSA, or full-thickness burns < 10% BSA.
Major: Partial-thickness burns > 20% BSA, full-thickness burns > 10%, or burns of special areas such as eyes, ears, hands, feet, and perineum.

Assess whether the mechanism of injury is consistent with the PE and development of the pt.
This assessment will help you decide whether to report possible neglect or abuse.

Differential diagnosis
Very few things can imitate a burn, but if you have what looks like a superficial burn (sunburn) and hypotension or shock, consider toxic shock syndrome or heat shock. Deeper burns are unlikely to be confused with anything else given the characteristic charring and other changes.

P **Specialized burn surgeons should manage pts with severe burns.**
Use the Parkland formula to calculate IV fluid requirements:
Parkland formula: Give 4 cc of Lactated ringer's or normal saline solution per kg body weight per % BSA burned over the first 24 hrs = 4 cc/kg/%BSA.
The first half should be given in the first 8 hrs from the time of injury and the second half in the next 16 hrs.
This fluid should be given in addition to the normal IV maintenance fluids.
On following days, D5LR or D5NS or 5% albumin may be used.

Place a Foley catheter to monitor urine output as a response to therapy.
Fluid should be titrated to a rate of 1 cc/kg/hr of urine output.

Check serum electrolytes and replace as needed.
There may be large changes and losses of electrolytes such as sodium and potassium because of the losses of fluid that occur with severe burns. If they are not replaced, the pt is at risk of potentially fatal sequelae such as arrhythmia, seizures, and cerebral edema.

Prevent infection with dressing changes and topical agents.
Dressings should be changed twice daily. Each dressing change should have a topical agent applied, such as Silvadene cream, Sulfamylon cream, or 1% Betadine.

Treat all fevers >37.5°C (99.5°F) with antipyretics and cooling measures, but only use antibiotics after cultures are positive and you have identified an organism.
Noninfectious fever occurs often with burns.

Nutrition
With a 40% BSA injury, children will have a 50% increase in energy expenditure.
Pay special attention to providing sufficient calories and vitamins, which can be provided by nasogastric tube if necessary.

Pain should be treated with IV narcotics.
Morphine sulfate with patient-controlled analgesia is effective.
Boluses should be given before dressing changes.

All pts with inhalation injuries should be intubated to protect their airway.

Index

CPSIA information can be obtained at www.ICGtesting.com
Printed in the USA
BVOW011353161112

305770BV00004B/5/A